BRAIN DOPAMINERGIC SYSTEMS: IMAGING WITH POSITRON TOMOGRAPHY

Developments in Nuclear Medicine

VOLUME 20

Series Editor: Peter H. Cox

The titles published in this series are listed at the end of this volume.

Brain Dopaminergic Systems: Imaging with Positron Tomography

Proceedings of a Workshop held in Caen, France
within the framework of the European Community
Medical and Public Health Research

edited by

J.C. BARON
INSERM U. 320, CYCERON, University of Caen, Caen, France

D. COMAR
E.E.C. Concerted Action on P.E.T. Investigations of Cellular Regeneration and Degeneration, Service Hospitalier Frédéric Joliot, Hôpital d'Orsay, Orsay, France

L. FARDE
Department of Psychiatry and Psychology, Karolinska Hospital, Stockholm, Sweden

J.L. MARTINOT
Service Hospitalier Frédéric Joliot, CEA-DRIPP Orsay, Paris-Sud University, Paris, France

and

B. MAZOYER
Service Hospitalier Frédéric Joliot, CEA-DRIPP Orsay, Paris-Sud University, Paris, France

SPRINGER SCIENCE+BUSINESS MEDIA, B.V.

ISBN 978-94-010-5561-1 ISBN 978-94-011-3528-3 (eBook)
DOI 10.1007/978-94-011-3528-3

Printed on acid-free paper

Softcover reprint of the hardcover 1st edition 1991

MEDICAL AND HEALTH RESEARCH PROGRAMME OF THE EC

BIOMEDICAL ENGINEERING IN THE EUROPEAN COMMUNITY

The involvement of the European Community (EC) in the field of Medical and Health Research started in 1978 with the first Programme which contained three projects. Since then, it has steadily expanded and it will include around 120 projects by the end of the fourth Programme (1987–1991).

The *general goal* of the programme is clearly to contribute to a better quality of life by improving health, and its *distinctive feature* is to strengthen European collaboration in order to achieve this goal.

The main objectives of this collaboration are:

- increase the *scientific efficiency* of the relevant research and development efforts in the Member States through their gradual coordination at Community level following the mobilization of the available research potential of national programmes, and also their *economic efficiency* through sharing of tasks and strengthening the joint use of available health research resources,
- *improve scientific and technological knowledge* in the research and development areas selected for their importance to all Member States, and promote its *efficient transfer into practical applications*, taking particular account of potential industrial and economic developments in the areas concerned,
- *optimize the capacity and economic efficiency of health care efforts* throughout the countries and regions of the Community.

The current programme consists of *six research targets*. Four are related to major health problems: CANCER, AIDS, AGE-RELATED PROBLEMS, and PERSONAL ENVIRONMENT AND LIFE-STYLE RELATED PROBLEMS; two are related to health resources: *MEDICAL TECHNOLOGY DEVELOPMENT* and HEALTH SERVICES RESEARCH.

Funds are provided by the Community for relevant "concerted action" activities which consist of research *COLLABORATION and COORDINATION* in EC Member States and/or in other European participant countries. *NETWORKS* of research institutes can be set up and supported by means of meetings, workshops, short-term staff exchanges/visits to other countries, information dissemination and so on; centralized facilities such as data banks, computing, and preparation and distribution of reference materials can also be funded. The funds are *not* direct research grants; the institutes concerned must fund the research activities carried out within their own countries – it is the international coordination activities which are eligible for Community support. Each such research network is placed under the responsibility of a *PROJECT LEADER* chosen from among the leading scientists in the network, with the assistance of a *PROJECT MANAGEMENT GROUP* representing the teams participating in the network.

The Commission of the European Communities is assisted in the execution of this programme by a Management and Coordination Advisory Committee (CGC – Medical and Health Research), and by Concerted Action Committees (COMACs) and Working Parties, composed of representatives and of scientific experts respectively, designated by the competent authorities of the Member States.

Other European countries, not belonging to the EC but participating in COST (Cooperation on Science and Technology) may take part in the Programme.

The present work was conducted according to the advice of *COMAC-BME* which supervises the coordination of research in *biomedical engineering* (BME) within the Medical Technology Development target.

More information may be obtained from: Commission of the European Communities
Directorate General XII-F-6
200 Rue de la Loi
B - 1049 Brussels

CONTENTS

PREFACE

Imaging of the Dopaminergic system in the human brain with the *in vivo* use of Positron Emission Tomography has emerged in the late 1980s as a tool of major importance in Clinical Neurosciences and Pharmacology. The last few years have witnessed the rapid development of new radiotracers specific to receptors, reuptake sites and enzymes of the dopamine system; the application of these radiotracers has led to major breakthroughs in the pathophysiology and therapy of movement disorders and schizophrenic-like psychoses. This book is the first to collect, in a single volume, state-of-the-art contributions to the various aspects of this research. Its contents address methodological issues related to the design, labelling, quantitative imaging and compartmental modelisation of radioligands of the post-synaptic, pre-synaptic and enzyme sites of the dopamine system and to their use in clinical research in the fields of Parkinson's disease as well as other movement disorders, psychoses and neuroleptic receptor occupancy. The chapters were written by leading European scientists in the field of Positron Emission Tomography, gathered together in Caen (France, November 1990) under the aegis of the EEC Concerted Action on "PET Investigations of Cellular Regeneration and Degeneration. This book provides a current and comprehensive overview on PET studies of the brain dopamine system which should aid and interest neurologists, psychiatrists, pharmacologists and medical imaging scientists.

J. C. Baron
D. Comar
L. Farde
J. L. Martinot
B. Mazoyer

August 1991

LIST OF CONTRIBUTORS

Dr Yves Agid
INSERM U 289
et Service de Neurologie et Neuropsychologie
Hôpital de la Salpêtrière
47, Bd de l'Hôpital
F-75651 PARIS Cédex 13
France

Dr J.C. Baron
INSERM U. 320, CYCERON
University of Caen
Boulevard H. Becquerel
P.O. Box 5027
F-14021 CAEN Cedex
France

Dr David J. Brooks
MRC Cyclotron Unit
Hammersmith Hospital
Ducane Road
LONDON W12 0HS
U.K.

Professor Dominique Comar
EEC Concerted Action on PET
Service Hospitalier Frédéric Joliot
Hôpital d'Orsay
F-91406 ORSAY
France

Dr R. de Beaurepaire
INSERM U. 320
Laboratoire de Pharmacologie
CHU Côte de Nacre
F-14032 CAEN
France

Dr L. Eriksson
Departments of Clinical Neurophysiology
and Neuroradiology
Karolinska Hospital
S-104 01 STOCKHOLM
Sweden

Co-authors: H. Herzog and A-L. Nordström

Dr L. Farde
Department of Psychiatry and Psychology
Karolinska Hospital
S-104 01 STOCKHOLM
Sweden

Dr C. Halldin
Department of Psychiatry and Psychology
Karolinska Hospital
S-104 01 STOCKHOLM
Sweden

Dr Philippe Hantraye
URA CNRS 1285, CEA, DSV
Service Hospitalier Frédéric Joliot
4 Place du Général Leclerc
F-91401 ORSAY Cédex
France

Dr K.L. Leenders
Paul Scherrer Institute
CH-5232 VILLIGEN
Switzerland

Dr J.L. Martinot
Service Hospitalier Frédéric Joliot, CEA
Hôpital d'Orsay
F-91406 ORSAY
France

Dr B.M. Mazoyer
Antenne d'Informatique Médicale
Hôpital Robert Debré
45 Boulevard Serrurier
F-75019 PARIS
France

Dr A-L. Nordström
Department of Psychiatry and Psychology
Karolinska Hospital
S-104 01 STOCKHOLM
Sweden

Dr E. Salmon
Department of Neurology and Cyclotron Research Center
University Hospital
Sart Tilman
B-4000 LIEGE
Belgium

Dr G. Stöcklin
Institute for Chemistry
Research Centre Jülich
P.O. Box 1913
DW-5170 JÜLICH
Germany

Dr J. Tedroff
Department of Neurology
Uppsala University
S-751 85 UPPSALA
Sweden

Co-authors: P. Hartvig, H. Ågren, P. Bjurling and B. Långström

Dr K. Wienhard
Max-Planck-Institute for Neurological Research
Gleueler Str. 50
DW-5000 COLOGNE 41
Germany

Dr S. Zijlstra
PET Center Groningen
University Hospital
Oostersingel 59
NL-9713 EZ GRONINGEN
The Netherlands

Co-authors: J.W. Louwerens, J.A. Buddingh, A.M.J. Paans, G. Visser, C.J. Slooff, W. Vaalburg and J. Korf

NEUROANATOMY OF DOPAMINERGIC SYSTEM IN THE HUMAN BRAIN

Yves AGID

Abstract. This introductory paper briefly describes the distribution of dopaminergic neuronal pathways and their main connexions in the human brain, with a special reference to Parkinson's disease.

Dopaminergic systems in human brain can be studied, in vivo, using positon emission tomography (PET). This can be done both at presynaptic level by visualizing the pattern of dopaminergic nerve terminals (fluorodopa uptake, dopamine uptake blockers) and at the postsynaptic level by measuring the density of dopaminergic receptors.

The pattern of distribution of dopaminergic neurons (around 300.000 on each side) in the human mesencephalon is heterogeneous. Within the substantia nigra pars compacta, their dendrites are interconnected horizontally whereas vertical dopaminergic dendrites running toward the substantia nigra pars reticulata receive nigral afferences from the striatum. For the sake of clarification, four dopaminergic neuronal groups can be described within the nigral complex in the human brain: the substantia nigra pars compacta which comprises three horizontal bands of dopaminergic cells (α, β, γ), the ventral tegmental area (corresponding to the A10 group in the rat), the peri- and retrorubral region (corresponding to the A8 region) and finally the central grey substance (near the acqueduc of Sylvius) (Graybiel et al 1990). One of the major differences between these neuronal groups is the proportion of pigmented-melanized neurons which varies from very high level for neurons in the substantia nigra pars compacta to intermediate level in the ventral tegmental area and A8 cell groups to very low level in dopaminergic neurons in the central grey substance (Hirsch et al 1988).

Dopaminergic fibers originating in the mesencephalon can be classified into three groups (Gerfen et al 1987). Fibers A and B contain dopamine, the former are thin, smooth with small varicosities, the latter being thicker with numerous large varicosities. Other larger dopaminergic fibers with voluminous varicosities (fibers C), however do not contain dopamine. Most of these dopaminergic neurons project towards the striatum known to have a compartmental architecture comprising of striosomes, identified as acetylcholinesterase-poor zones and extrastriosomal matrix. The projections from striosomes is back towards the substantia nigra pars compacta whereas the extra-striosomal matrix projects massively to the pallidum and the substantia nigra pars reticulata. The dopaminergic innervation of the striatum is denser in the matrix than in striosomes (Graybiel et al 1987). Within the striatum, fibers A are mainly distributed in the matrix, fibers B in the striosomes, fibers C being more diffusely distributed. In addition, the striatal projections of the dopaminergic terminals can be also distinguished according to their origin in the mesencephalon: a) those

J. C. Baron et al. (eds.), Brain Dopaminergic Systems: Imaging with Positron Tomography, 1–4.

issued from the ventral tegmental area innervate the ventral striatum; b) those from the substantia nigra pars compacta (dorsal and ventral part) project towards the matrix of the dorsolateral striatum and the striosomes of the dorsomedian striatum, respectively; and c) neurones from the A8 area are directed towards the matrix of the dorsal striatum (Jimenez Castellanos and Graybiel 1987). Such distinctions between the dopaminergic innervation of the matrix and striosomes in the striatum have functional implications. Striosomes and matrix are enriched in dopaminergic D1 and D2 receptors, respectively (Besson et al 1988). The striato-nigral system can be divided into two different outputs (Gerfen et al 1990). a) A direct striato-nigral system which inhibits the substantia nigra, is modulated by striatal dopaminergic afferences through dopaminergic D1 receptors. b) An indirect striato-pallido-subthalamo-nigral output is modulated by nigrostriatal dopaminergic nerve terminals essentially through dopaminergic D2 receptors. In brief, the selective stimulation of striatal D1 and D2 dopaminergic receptors seem to trigger two main striatal outputs: one which, is direct and inhibitory, is stimulated by dopaminergic fibers; the other, which is indirect and excitatory, is inhibited by dopaminergic fibers. In normal conditions, the sum of these two nigrostriatal dopaminergic activities reinforce the activation of the striato-nigro-thalamo-cortical circuit. In Parkinson's disease, degeneration of the nigrostriatal dopaminergic pathway leads to inhibition of the above described complex loop (Alexander and Crutcher 1990). However, such an interpretation is partially misleading for two reasons. The description of two separate striato-nigral systems is probably too rigid considering that there is only a relative predominance of identified dopaminergic neurones and of D1 and D2 dopaminergic receptors within striosomes and extrastriosomal matrix. Secondly and perhaps more importantly, in Parkinson's disease, the degeneration of dopaminergic neurons is variable from one patient to another and according to the course of the disease. It is much more complex than previously described (Agid et al 1989). Following points can be made as to the nature of the complexity.

a) Within the ventral mesencephalon, not all dopamine-containing neurons are damaged: the heavily melanized cell groups seem to be more vulnerable.

b) The nigrostriatal dopaminergic system is more severely affected (90 %) than the mesocorticolimbic (50 %) system.

c) Within the striatum, there is a gradient loss of dopaminergic fibers, the greatest deficit occurring dorso-laterally both in the caudate nucleus and in the putamen, the ventro-medial part of the striatum being relatively spared.

d) The surviving nigrostriatal dopamine-containing neurons become overactive as a function of the severity of the lesion, this mechanism of compensation which has not been demonstrated in the mesocorticolimbic dopaminergic system.

e) The density of dopaminergic D1 and D2 binding sites in the striatum (putamen and caudate nucleus) is not dramatically changed. Nevertheless, the following conclusions still remain controversial or unproven: the density of dopamine binding sites is increased in striatal areas (putamen) where dopamine depletion exceeds 90 % ; levodopa and bromocriptine treatments tend to decrease the density of dopaminergic D2 binding sites ; levodopa-induced dyskinesia are seen in patients with increased striatal D1 and D2 receptors. In the substantia nigra the densities of dopamine D2 and D1 binding sites are decreased and unaltered, respectively. This is at variance from what is observed in progressive supranuclear palsy, a parkinsonian syndrome which does not respond to long-term levodopa treatment: the density of striatal D2 dopamine receptors is decreased, as shown in vitro and in vivo using PET, whereas D1 receptors seem to be unchanged.

f) It is generally assumed that the first parkinsonian symptom appears when at least 70% of the nigrostriatal system is damaged.

g) The striatal "dopamine deficiency syndrome" is a characteristic of parkinsonian disorders, including post-encephalic and MPTP-induced parkinsonism (with a dramatic response to levodopa), progressive supranuclear palsy and multiple system atrophies (with little and no response to levodopa).

In conclusion, what do we expect from PET studies in order to assess the dopaminergic functions in the brain of parkinsonian patients? a) longitudinal evaluation of the slow and progressive loss of striatal dopaminergic neurons during the course of the disease (linear? polynomial? exponential?) in the various parkinsonian syndromes; b) search for correlations between pattern and severity of the loss of nigrostriatal dopaminergic neurons and parkinsonian symptoms as well as levodopa-induced side effects; c) study of the pattern of distribution and especially of density of striatal dopaminergic receptors (D1 to D5) in an attempt to approach the pathophysiological mechanism of levodopa-induced dyskinesia, of fluctuations of performances, and of mental disturbances; d) estimation of the survival of foetal dopaminergic neurons (genetically engineered dopaminergic cells ?) grafted in the striatum of parkinsonian patients. There are only few of the questions that can now be examined.

References :

Graybiel, A.M., Hirsch E.C., Agid Y. (1990) 'The nigrostriatal system in Parkinson's disease', in 9th International Symposium on Parkinson's disease. Jerusalem, June 5-9. M.B. Streifler, A.D. Korczyn, E. Melamed, M.B. Youdim (eds.) Raven Press, New York, 53, 17-20.

Hirsch E.C., Graybiel A.M., Agid Y. (1988) 'Melanized dopaminergic neurons are differentially susceptible to degeneration in Parkinson's disease', Nature, 334, 6180, 345-348.

Gerfen C.R., Herkenham M., Thibault J (1987) 'The neostriatal mosaic: II. Patch-and matrix-directed mesostriatal dopaminergic and non-dopaminergic systems', J. Neurosci., 7, 3915-3934.

Graybiel A.M., Hirsch E.C., Agid Y. (1987) 'Differences in tyrosine hydroxylase-like immunoreactivity characterize the mesostriatal innervation of striosomes and extrastriosomal matrix at maturity', P.N.A.S., 84, 303-307.

Jimenez Castellanos J.and Graybiel A.M. (1987) 'Subdivisions of the dopamine-containing A8-A9-A10 complex identified by their differential mesostriatal innervation of striosomes and extrastriosomal matrix', Neurosc., 23, 223-242.

Besson M.J., Graybiel A.M., Nastuk M. (1988) '(3H)SCH 23390 binding to D1 dopamine receptors in the basal ganglia of the cat and primate: delineation of striosomal compartments and pallidal and nigral subdivisions', Neurosc., 26, 101-119.

Gerfen C.R., Thomas M.E., Lawrence C.M., ZVI S., Thomas N.C., Frederick J.M., David R.S. (1990) 'D1 and D2 dopamine receptor-regulated gene expression of striatonigral and striatopallidal neurons, Science, 250, 1429-1432.

Alexander G.E. and Crutcher M.D. (1990) 'Functional architecture of basal ganglia circuits: neural substrates of parallel processing. TINS, 13, 266-271.

Agid Y., Cervera P., Hirsch E.C., Javoy-Agid F., Lehericy S., Raisman R., Ruberg M. (1989) 'Biochemistry of Parkinson's disease 28 years later: a critical review'. Mov. Disord., 4 (suppl. 1), 126-144.

RADIOLIGANDS FOR PET STUDIES OF D_2-RECEPTORS: BUTYROPHENONE AND ERGOT DERIVATIVES

G. STÖCKLIN

ABSTRACT. Chemical and pharmacological aspects of various butyrophenone neuroleptics and of bromolisuride are reviewed with respect to their suitability for PET studies of dopaminergic receptors.

INTRODUCTION

Butyrophenone neuroleptics are most widely used for PET studies of D_2-receptors. The reason for their wide application and evaluation as PET tracers is that their binding properties are generally well established, and that these dopamine antagonists exhibit a high selective affinity to the D_2-receptor. The 4(p-fluorophenyl)-4-oxobutylamino structure required for cerebral dopaminergic receptor binding (Janssen 1973) is common to all butyrophenone neuroleptics (Fig. 1) and is considered to be the pharmacophore, although even the introduction of the large iodine atom in the 2'-position of the fluorobenzene ring of the pharmacophore hardly changes the binding properties (Saji et al 1986).

Among the synthetic ergoline compounds such as lergotrile, pergolide, bromocryptine and lisuride only the brominated lisuride has been used for PET. While lisuride is a dopamine agonist, bromolisuride has been shown to be an antagonist (Wachtel et al 1983).

In this paper chemical and pharmacological aspects of the D_2-ligands which have been evaluated for PET studies will be reviewed.

CHOICE OF RADIONUCLIDE

Butyrophenone neuroleptics have been labelled with the positron emitters ^{11}C ($T_{½}$ = 20 min), ^{18}F ($T_{½}$ = 110 min), ^{75}Br ($T_{½}$ = 96 min) and ^{76}Br ($T_{½}$ = 16 h) in various positions (Fig. 1). Also several γ-emitting radionuclides have been used. Planar γ-ray imaging using spiroperidol labelled at the non-essential aniline moiety with bromine-77 was the first study performed (Friedman et al 1982, Crawley et al 1984). Bromine-77, however, is a poor radionuclide for SPECT, PET, and planar imaging, due to its high γ-energies. The butyrophenone neuroleptics all contain a fluorine atom at the pharmacophore and thus lend themselves to labelling with fluorine-18 without changing the molecule. Some of the first studies have used this approach (Tewson et al 1980, Welch et al 1983, Arnett et al 1985a). Recently an easier direct fluorination procedure has become

J. C. Baron et al. (eds.), Brain Dopaminergic Systems: Imaging with Positron Tomography, 5–22.

available (Hamacher et al 1986, 1991). Carbon-11 has first been used successfully in ^{11}C-methylation of the amido group of spiroperidol (Wagner et al 1983). N-Methylspiroperidol (MSP) has an even higher affinity to the D_2-receptor than spiroperidol itself, however, the half life of carbon-11 is somewhat short for measuring the relatively slow kinetics of these irreversible butyrophenone ligands.

As a longer-lived alternative to ^{11}C-alkylation, fluoroalkylation of the amido group of spiroperidol, e.g. N-[^{18}F]fluoroethylspiroperidol has also been evaluated (Coenen et al 1987a, Chi et al 1986, Shiue et al 1987, Satyamurthy et al 1986). Labelling of the anilino ring at the nonessential part of the molecule with the positron emitters bromine-75 and bromine-76 was also applied (Maziere et al 1984, Moerlein et al 1986). Bromine-75 with 1.6 h half life decays with only 75% β^+ and has a very abundant 287 keV γ-line which is emitted with a 1.3 nsec delay after β^+-emission. Bromine-76 with 16 h half life has only 57% β^+-emission and also a very abundant γ-line of 559 keV which is emitted with a 12 psec delay after the β^+-emission. These γ-lines of ^{75}Br and ^{76}Br can give rise to randoms. Also the β^+-energy of ^{76}Br is fairly high with 3.4 MeV. In Table 1 the radiation doses to target organs are given for ^{75}Br- and ^{76}Br-labelled spiroperidol (Sp) as extrapolated from studies with bromine-77 (Crawley et al 1984). Doses are also given for N-[^{18}F]fluoroethylspiroperidol (FESP) and for ^{18}F-labelled spiroperidol itself. The studies with [^{18}F]FESP were carried out with a whole body PET in humans (Herzog et al 1990), those of [^{18}F]Sp were extrapolated from rat studies (Welch et al 1988). It can be seen that the doses from the ^{75}Br- and in particular those from the ^{76}Br-labelled ligands are considerably higher than those for the ^{18}F-labelled molecules. Since bromine-75 cannot be prepared free from the longer-lived bromine-76 the actual doses for the ^{75}Br-labelled ligands are also significantly higher than shown in Table 1. Since the kinetics and biodistribution of [^{76}Br]bromolisuride are similar to those of [^{76}Br]Sp, the radiation doses should also be comparable.

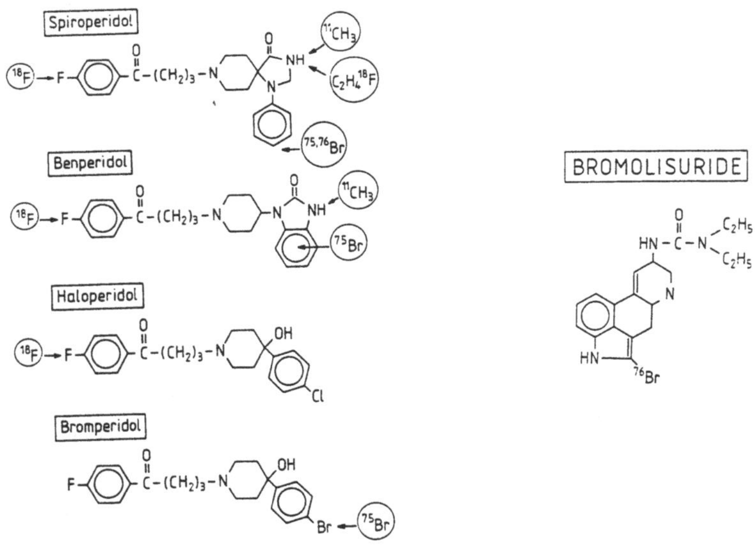

Fig. 1 Positron-emitter labelled butyrophenone neuroleptics and bromolisuride

Both ^{75}Br and ^{76}Br require a medium energy cyclotron for production (for a review cf. Qaim 1986). In addition to the relatively high radiation doses the binding properties of these brominated ligands are also not ideal (see below).

Table 1 Radiation dose to target organs from ^{75}Br- and ^{76}Br-bromospiroperidol and from N-^{18}F-fluoroethylspiroperidol. μGy/MBq (mrad/mCi)

	^{75}Br-Sp [1]	^{76}Br-Sp [1]	^{18}F-FESP [2]	^{18}F-Sp [3]
Adrenals	22.4(83)	316.2(1170)	17.0(63)	
Bladder wall	38.4(142)	537.8(1990)	83.2(308)	
Kidneys	20.3(75)	275.7(1020)	13.2(49)	18.1(67)
Liver	140.5(520)	1632.4(6040)	65.9(244)	7.3(27)
Lungs	110.8(410)	1178.4(4360)	9.5(35)	7.6(28)
Marrow (red)	15.9(59)	201.1(744)	10.0(37)	13.0(48)
Muscle	13.5(50)	191.4(708)	10.0(37)	12.4(46)
Ovaries	13.2(49)	239.7(887)	10.8(40)	
Pancreas	20.5(76)	291.9(1080)	14.6(54)	
Spleen	16.3(60)	205.4(760)	9.7(36)	140.5(520)
Gallbladder	?	?	207.3(767)	?
Total body	18.6(69)	243.8(902)	11.9(44)	13.0(48)

[1] Crawley et al 1984 (man, γ-camera), extrapolated from ^{77}Br-Sp.
[2] Herzog et al 1990 (man, PET)
[3] Welch et al 1988 (rats)

SYNTHETIC ASPECTS

^{11}C-Methylation of the amido group of spiroperidol is a relatively easy procedure. An improved synthesis of (3-N-[^{11}C]methyl)spiroperidol (MSP) has been described (Dannals et al 1986). Important is to obtain high specific activities in the order of 1,000 mCi/μmole at the end of synthesis. N-^{11}C-methylbenperidol has recently also been prepared and evaluated (Suehiro et al 1990).

The n.c.a. introduction of fluorine-18 into butyrophenone neuroleptics was achieved via the labelled precursor p-[^{18}F]fluorobenzonitril in a multi-step synthesis with radiochemical yields of 10-20% within 90 minutes (Shiue et al 1985). This method is superior to the triazene decomposition used earlier (Welch et al 1983) which only gives rise to poor radiochemical yields. Recently a direct nucleophilic ^{18}F-for-NO_2 exchange was accomplished on the p-nitro-desfluoro-N-methylspiroperidol precursor (Hamacher et al

1986, 1991). The problem in this aminopolyether promoted nucleophilic reaction (Fig. 2) lies in the basic conditions which have to be carefully buffered by oxalate to avoid enolization of the ketone function (Gysemans and Mertens 1990) and major destruction of the precursor.

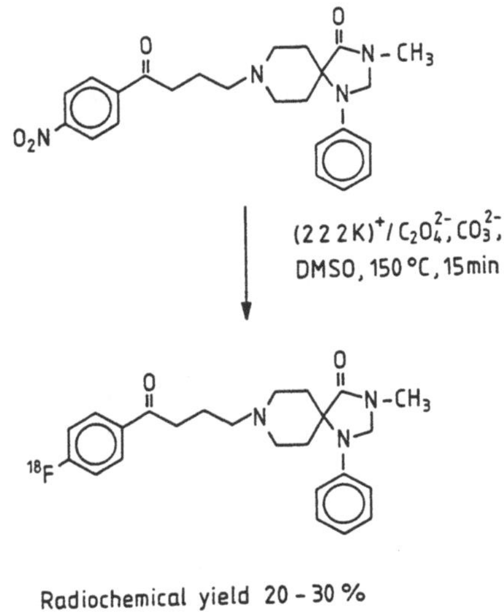

Fig. 2 Direct nucleophilic fluorination of [^{18}F]MSP (Hamacher et al 1991)

A general problem is specific activity or rather effective specific activity. The effective specific activity is also related to impurities other than the cold target molecule itself. In the case of [^{18}F]methylspiroperidol prepared by the synthesis described in Fig. 2, decomposition products can be eliminated by solid change extraction of the product on a cartridge containing a cation exchanger on silica gel (Hamacher et al 1991). Radiochemical yields of 15-20% are obtained and specific activities ≥ 1,000 mCi/μmole.

Since the direct nucleophilic fluorination in the original position of the butyrophenone neuroleptic itself was not achievable for some time, various groups focused on the fluoroalkylation of spiroperidol, starting with disubstituted [^{18}F]fluoroalkanes which are prepared by nucleophilic ^{18}F-fluorination of halogen-, tosyl-, or triflyl-groups (Block et al 1986, 1987; Chi et al 1986; Satyamurthy et al 1986; Shiue et al 1987). A reaction scheme is shown in Fig. 3 for the synthesis of [^{18}F]FESP.

Most investigators perform fluoride exchange and subsequent condensation with spiroperidol in a one-pot mode. It was, however, observed that under the basic conditions used (Kryptofix/K_2CO_3 or $R_4N^+OH^-$), cold fluoride is released from the spiroperidol thus lowering the specific activity. It was therefore recommended to separate the [^{18}F]fluoroalkyl intermediate from its cold disubstituted precursor to ensure high specific activity (Coenen et al 1987a, 1989) even though the overall radiochemical yield is then only 15-20%, and a synthesis time of 60 minutes is required.

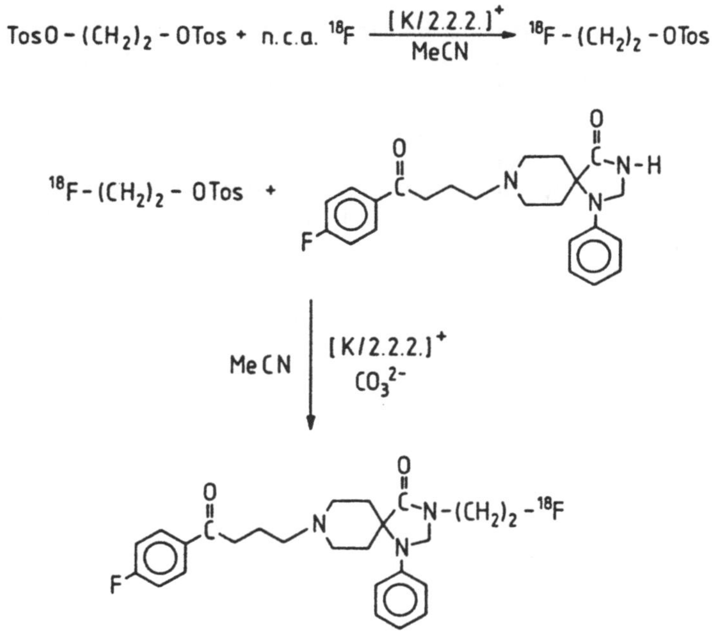

Fig. 3 [^{18}F]Fluoroethylation of N-methylspiroperidol

A variety of radiobrominated butyrophenone neuroleptics has been prepared as mentioned above. Electrophilic bromination of the anilino ring can easily be achieved by in-situ oxidation of radiobromide (for reviews cf. Coenen et al 1983 and Mazière and Loc'h 1986a). Best suited for in-situ oxidation with high yields and little by-products is hydrogen peroxide in glacial acetic acid, i.e. peracetic acid (Moerlein et al 1988). [^{75}Br]Bromperidol was prepared by regiospecific bromination via destannylation of the tin precursor using H_2O_2/CH_3COOH with radiochemical yields of 35% in 30 minutes and a specific activity of 10^4 mCi/µmole (Moerlein and Stöcklin 1985). A variety of radiobrominated spiroperidol and alkylated spiroperidol molecules has been prepared by in-situ oxidation using either dichloramine-T or hydrogen peroxide-glacial acetic acid as in-situ oxidants, similar to the first studies by DeJesus et al (1983). Radiobromination of the 2-position of the indol ring of lisuride has also been achieved by this method with 60% radiochemical yield within 20 minutes (Loc'h and Mazière 1989b).

METABOLISM; FATE OF THE LABEL

Metabolism of the ligand, i.e. the fate of the label is essential for any modelling and quantitation since PET cannot distinguish between the individual ^{18}F-species. Metabolism at the site of action as well as in the periphery must be known. The fraction of unchanged ligand is important also in arterial blood with respect to the input function. Metabolite analysis in tissue and blood of small animals is the first step which requires elaborate radioanalytical studies and is mainly done by radiochromatography.

Analysis of brain tissue can be carried out by simple extraction of the homogenized tissue with methanol followed by HPLC analysis. This has been done for [^{18}F]FESP (Coenen et al 1987a) and for [^{18}F]MSP (Arnett et al 1985b). In the case of [^{18}F]MSP it was demonstrated that in the striatum of rats 98% was present as unchanged ligand even after 4 hours while in the cerebellum it was 90 and 85% of the extracted activity after 1 and 4 hours, respectively. If there are no differences in metabolism of this radioligand between rat and primate brain, then one may assume negligible contribution from radioactive metabolites during PET studies of [^{18}F]MSP. Also in the case of [^{18}F]haloperidol HPLC analysis of mouse brain homogenates at 30 and 60 minutes after injection showed that 95% of the radioactivity was intact tracer (Schlyer et al 1991) in agreement with metabolic studies with [^{14}C]haloperidol (Miyazaki et al 1986). The biodegradation of butyrophenone neuroleptics proceeds via oxidative N-dealkylation (Soudijn et al 1967) as shown in Fig. 4.

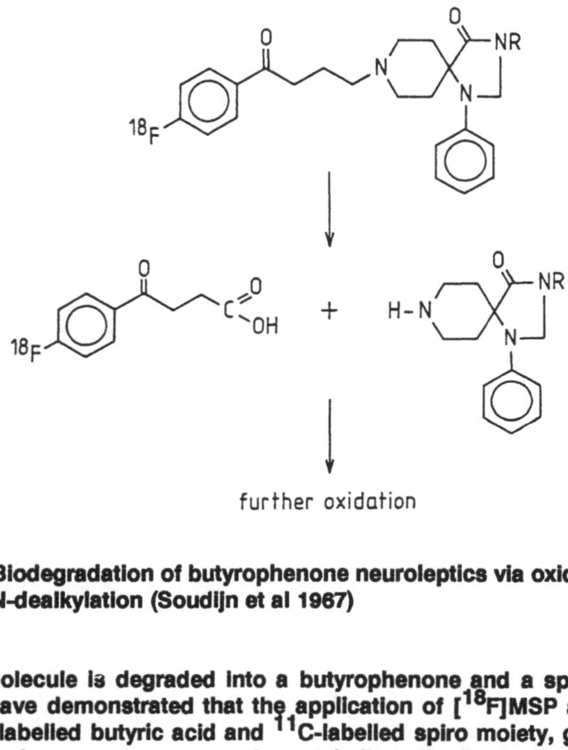

Fig. 4 Biodegradation of butyrophenone neuroleptics via oxidative N-dealkylation (Soudijn et al 1967)

The molecule is degraded into a butyrophenone and a spiro component. Fowler et al (1986) have demonstrated that the application of [^{18}F]MSP and N-[^{11}C]MSP, leading to the ^{18}F-labelled butyric acid and ^{11}C-labelled spiro moiety, gives rise to almost identical plasma clearance curves and metabolite distribution. If unidentified ^{11}C-labelled metabolites are produced in the brain or are delivered to the brain by plasma, their effect is small, since they do not measurably affect uptake and egress of radioactivity from striatum and cerebellum as determined by PET.

Blood analysis can be directly carried out by HPLC of the heparinized plasma. In general, the radioactivity in blood decreases rapidly in the first few minutes after i.v. injection of the radioligand. This is shown in Fig. 5 for [^{18}F]FESP, in which case the unchanged ligand decreases to about 10% after 3 hours in baboon brain, in human brain

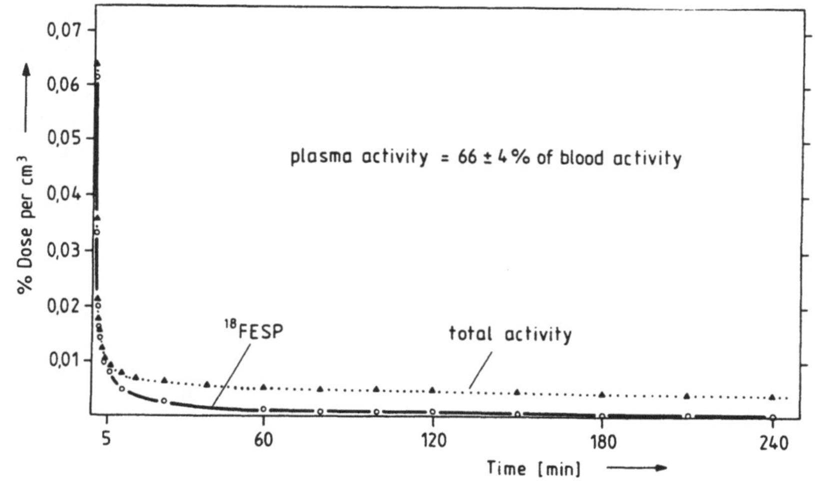

Fig. 5 Time course of ^{18}F-radioactivity and unchanged ligand in baboon plasma after i.v. injection of [^{18}F]FESP (Coenen et al 1988b)

to only about 55% (Wienhard et al 1990). This rapid blood clearance is almost identical in the case of [^{18}F]MSP (Fowler et al 1986).

Bromolisuride (BLIS) is a relatively stable molecule. Its metabolism is well known (Fig. 6). It occurs via hydrolysis at the urea moiety, hydroxylation at the benzene ring, and debromination (Loc'h et al 1989a).

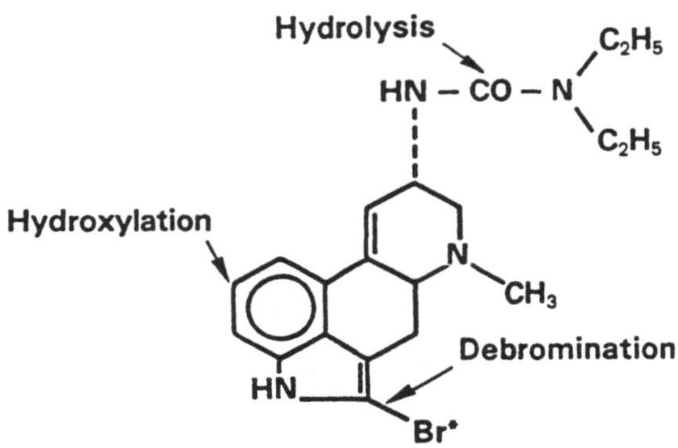

Fig. 6 Metabolism of ^{76}Br-bromolisuride (Loc'h et al 1989a)

Post mortem analyses in baboon brains 3 hours after i.v. injection shows that 83% of the radioactivity in the striatum and 52% in the cerebellum is present as unchanged BLIS (Mazière et al 1986b).

For [^{76}Br]BLIS, an elaborate analytical procedure has been developed which also allows to distinguish between bound and free ligands (Mazière et al 1990). In the case of the longer lived radionuclides such as bromine-75,76 and fluorine-18 this is possible despite the small activity levels. It is, however, hardly applicable to carbon-11.

PHARMACOKINETICS, UPTAKE AND SELECTIVITY

For the application of D_2-radioligands in PET studies, uptake and selectivity are important features. All butyrophenone neuroleptics are so-called irreversible ligands, i.e. dissociation from the receptor site is almost negligible. The regional cerebral pharmacokinetics of four different spiroperidol tracers as measured by PET in baboons are shown in Fig. 7.

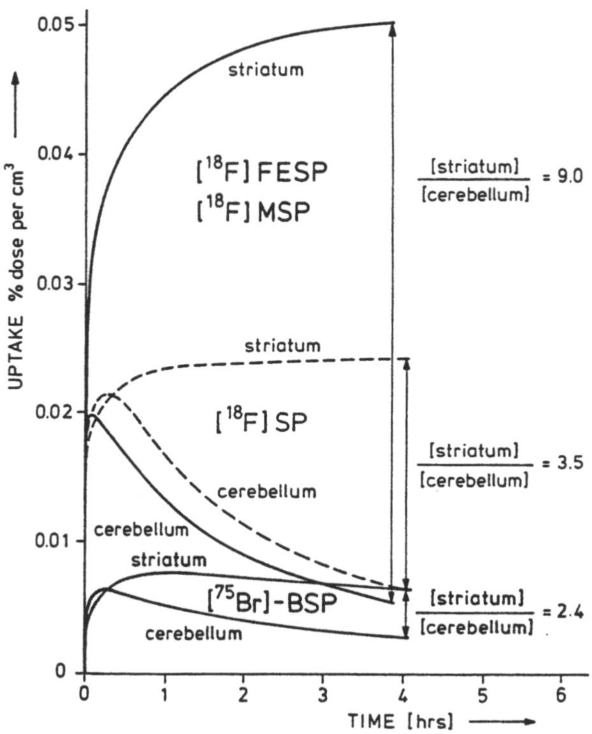

Fig. 7 Uptake and striatum-to-cerebellum ratio of FESP, MSP, SP and BSP in baboon brain (data taken from Coenen et al 1988b; Arnett et al 1985b; Moerlein et al 1986)

The highest striatal uptake is observed for [^{18}F]MSP and [^{18}F]FESP. These two ligands also exhibit the highest ratio striatum-to-cerebellum (about 9.0), which is considerably higher than for spiperone, [^{18}F]SP, itself (about 3.5). Spiperone labelled in the aniline ring with bromine-75 shows the lowest uptake and selectivity. It is clear from Fig. 7 that the ligands of choice are [^{18}F]MSP or [^{18}F]FESP, since they provide the highest sensitivity and the best contrast for PET studies. All ligands exhibit a saturation concentration in the striatum, which remains constant over many hours.

Neuroleptics are transported across the blood-brain barrier due to their high lipophilicity. However, when the lipophilicity of the ligands is plotted against the striatal uptake and the striatum-to-cerebellum ratio, no general trend is observed (Fig. 8). While MSP and FESP have a higher lipophilicity than SP and accordingly show a higher uptake, this is no longer true for bromospiperone (BSP), bromperidol (BP) and brombenperidol (BBP), which exhibit a very low uptake despite their high lipophilicity. Also the selectivity in terms of striatum-to-cerebellum ratio (4 hours p.i.) does not show any trend, either with respect to lipophilicity or with respect to K_D values.

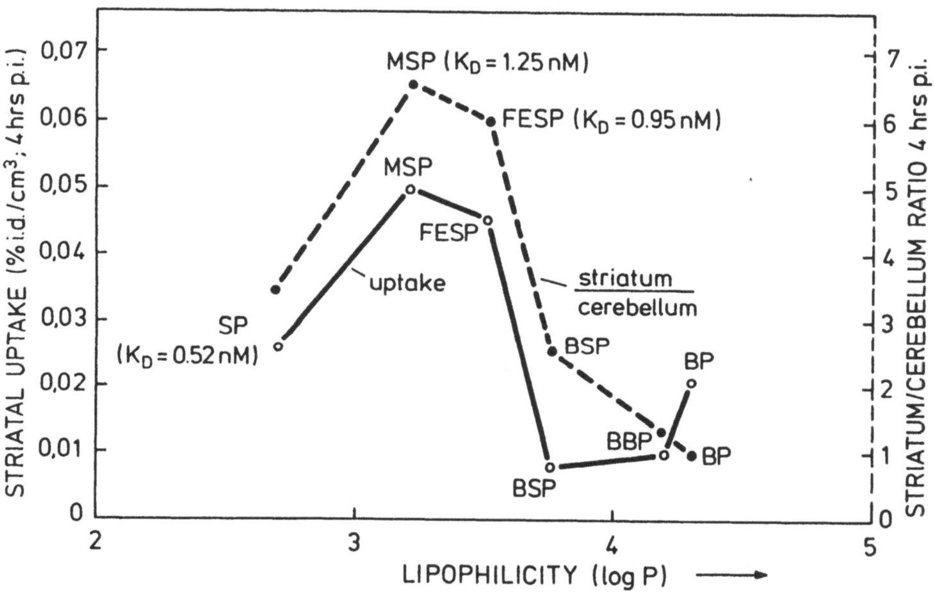

Fig. 8 Uptake and striatum-to cerebellum ratio in baboon as a function of lipophilicity for various butyrophenone neuroleptics (data taken from Coenen et al 1988b; Arnett et al 1985a; Moerlein et al 1986)

Another interesting feature of irreversibly binding ligands as demonstrated in the case of FESP (Coenen et al 1987b), is the fact that it can hardly be displaced, particularly at later times p.i.. Fig. 9 shows an almost negligible effect when displacement (by a 5,000 fold excess of the cold ligand) is done at 2 hours p.i. (upper curves). However, when the displacement is done 20 min p.i. (lower curves) about 50% can be displaced. The time dependence of the extent of displacibility cannot be explained by the dissociation kinetics, and the question remains whether this kind of irreversibility is due to internalization (Chugani et al 1988). The fact that the extent of displacibility decreases with time p.i seems to indicate that if some kind of internalization occurs, it is a relatively slow process which proceeds with a half time of about 20 minutes in the case of FESP.

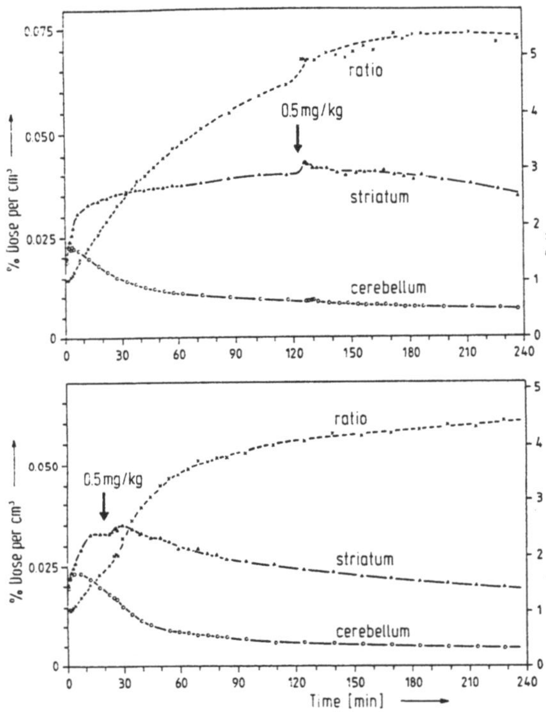

Fig. 9 Pharmacokinetics and displacement of [^{18}F]FESP by 0,5 mg/kg cold FESP 20 min p.i. (lower curve) and 2 hours p.i. in baboon brain as measured with PET (Coenen et al 1987b)

BLIS, on the other hand, is a reversible ligand, as can be seen from Fig. 10. The cerebral uptake of [^{76}Br]BLIS in baboon passes through a maximum at about 30 minutes (upper curves), and displacement by haloperidol is almost complete after 6 hours (lower curves).

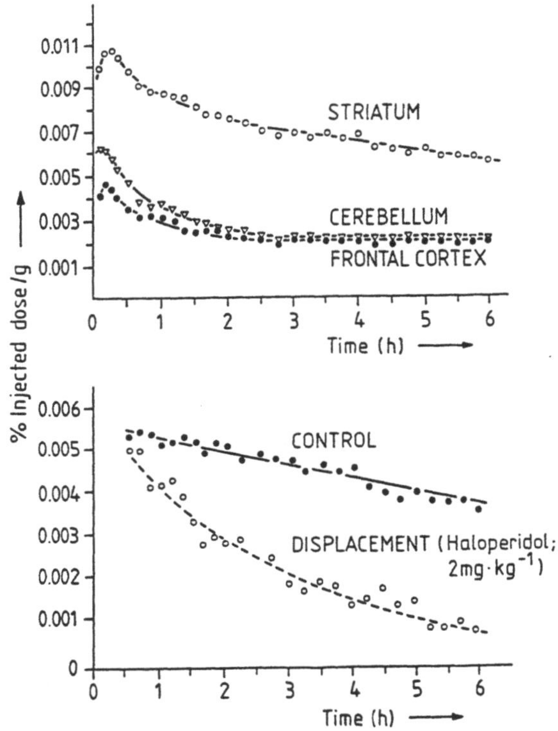

Fig. 10 Pharmacokinetics and displacement of [^{76}Br]BLIS by 2 mg/kg haldol in baboon brain as measured with PET (Mazière et al 1986b)

A further problem is the binding to receptors other than D_2, e.g. to S_2 receptors. For FESP this fraction is small (Fig. 11). The ratio frontal cortex-to-cerebellum is only 1.5 compared to 8.7 for the striatum-to-cerebellum ratio (Coenen et al 1988b). In baboon the binding of FESP in S_2-tissue is only about 10 to 20% of the D_2-binding. This is without correction of unspecific binding! Fig. 11 also shows that N-[^{18}F]propylspiroperidol ([^{18}F]FPSP) exhibits a lower uptake and a higher frontal cortex-to-cerebellum ratio than [^{18}F]FESP.

The Gjedde-Patlack plot for [^{18}F]FESP in man is shown in Fig. 12 (Wienhard et al 1990). While for the caudate and the pituitary the curves eventually approach a straight line with a positive slope, indicating irreversible binding, the cerebellum exhibits a horizontal curve, indicating that the tissue activity equilibrates with blood activity, and that there is no specific binding. Cortex shows a very small positive slope according to the small contribution from S_2-binding.

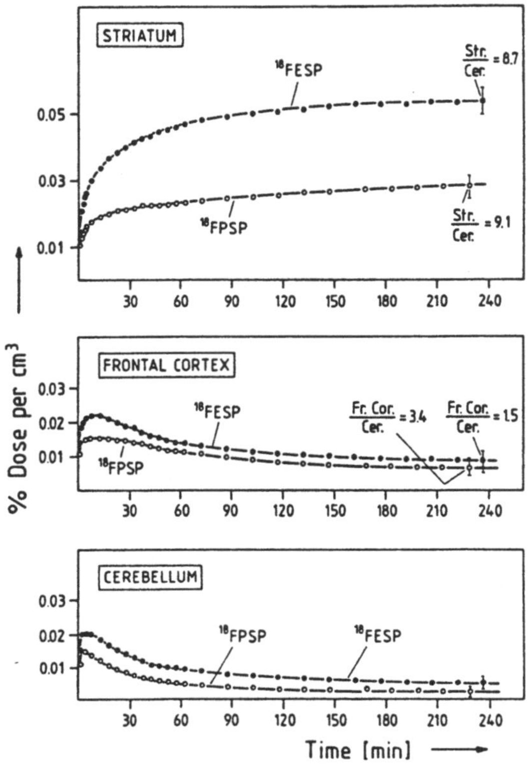

Fig. 11 Comparison of regional cerebral pharmacokinetics of [^{18}F]FESP and [^{18}F]FSP in baboon as measured with PET (Coenen et al 1988b)

More recently N-[^{11}C]methylbenperidol (NMB) was prepared and evaluated in mice and baboon (Suehiro et al 1990). A high striatal-to-cerebellar ratio of 11 was obtained at 60 minutes after injection. The authors claim on the basis of mice experiments that [^{11}C]NMB is a reversible ligand. On the other hand, their baboon data indicate no decrease of caudate tracer concentration at 100 minutes after injection. In any case NMB is a highly selective ligand for the D_2 receptor with an almost complete lack of S_2-receptor binding in the striatum.

Also the reversible ligand bromolisuride exhibits a very selective binding to D_2 receptors as demonstrated by in vivo competition experiments in rat brain (Mazière et al 1986b).

Some butyrophenone neuroleptics seem to exhibit extensive binding to other than D_2-receptor sites. This has also been demonstrated by PET in primates: Bromperidol (BP), a clinically used neuroleptic shows higher or identical binding to the cerebellum when compared with the striatum (Moerlein et al 1986). As shown in Fig. 13, both striatum and cerebellum activity concentration continue to increase even 2 hours after injection of [^{85}Br]bromperidol. This is also true for [^{75}Br]brombenperidol (BBP), in which case

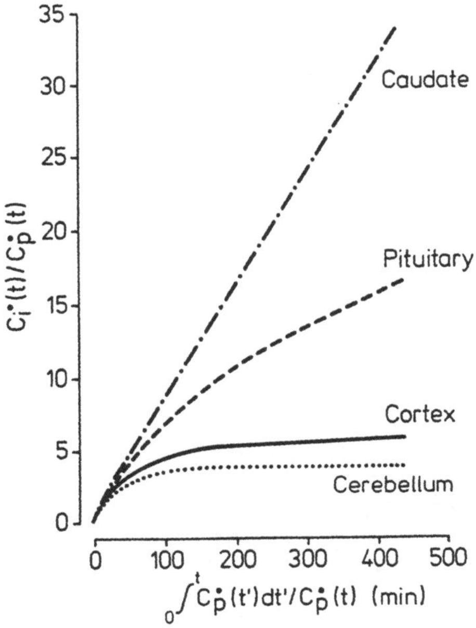

Fig. 12 Gjedde-Patlak plot of regional brain activity in humans after injection of [^{18}F]FESP (Wienhard et al 1990)

cerebellar activity is only slightly lower than the striatal activity; both do not show any decrease 160 minutes after injection, while [^{75}Br]bromspiroperidol (BSP) passes through a maximum at about 1 hour after injection; the slow decrease in both cerebellum and striatum proceeds with an almost identical slope. The kinetics of these brominated ligands, in particular the continued increase of cerebellum and striatum activity of BP and BBP seems to indicate that the transport kinetics of the tracer from plasma to brain is relatively slow compared to the receptor binding or other binding mechanisms in which case blood flow would significantly contribute to the observed kinetics. The high retention of activity in the cerebellum may also reflect binding to other receptor types such as σ-opioide receptors (Schlyer et al 1991).

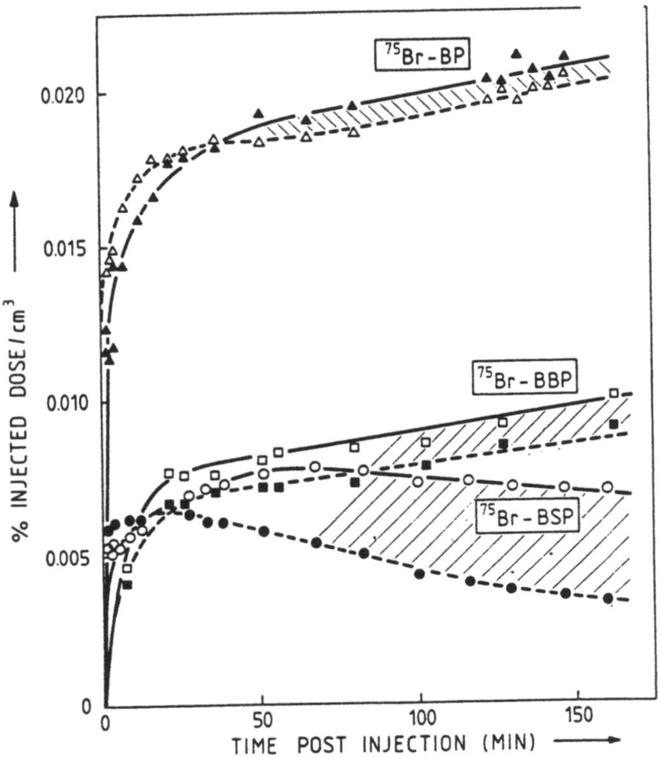

Fig. 13 Regional cerebral pharmacokinetics of ^{75}Br-labelled butyrophenone neuroleptics in baboon, as determined with PET. Empty symbols are for the striatum, filled symbols for the cerebellum (Moerlein et al 1986)

Similar effects are observed with [^{18}F]haloperidol in humans (Schlyer et al 1991). Minimal clearance of fluorine-18 activity from the brain was observed during a 10 hour period of the study. The regional cerebral distribution of this PET-study was consistent with post mortem measurements of σ-receptor density except for the basal ganglia and thalamus (Weissmann et al 1988).

^{18}F-Labelled butyrophenone neuroleptics have also been used to measure D_2-receptor occupancy by PET and to correlate haldol plasma levels with the D_2-receptor occupancy in the striatum (Smith et al 1988, Wolkin et al 1989). Central D_2-receptor blockade by neuroleptics has also been studied with [^{76}Br]bromospiroperidol (Baron et al 1989) and [^{76}Br]lisuride (Martinot et al 1990).

CONCLUSION

Among the butyrophenone neuroleptics both [^{18}F]MSP and [^{18}F]FESP seem to be the most useful ligands for PET studies of D_2-receptors. They are sufficiently selective for D_2-sites, show high uptake and suitable metabolic stability. the half life of fluorine-18 is compatible with the relatively slow cerebral pharmacokinetics. Chemical synthesis is relatively easy, particularly when considering the new direct nucleophilic fluorination for labelling of [^{18}F]MSP. Both MSP and FESP are irreversible ligands. [^{75}Br]BLIS, on the other hand, is a reversible ligand with high selectivity for the D_2-receptor and suitable metabolic stability. Its chemical synthesis is extremely easy. However, the poor availability of bromine-75,76, and the relatively high radiation doses to target organs are disadvantageous.

REFERENCES

Arnett, C.D., Shiue, C.-Y., Wolf, A.P., Fowler, J.S., Logan, J., and Watanabe, M. (1985a) 'Comparison of three ^{18}F-labeled butyrophenone neuroleptics drugs in the baboon using positron emission tomography', J. Neurochem. 44, 835.

Arnett, C.D., Fowler, J.S., Wolf, A.P., Shiue, C.-Y., and McPerson, D.W. (1985b) '[^{18}F]N-methylspiperone: The radioligand of choice for PET studies of the dopamine receptor in human brain', Life Sci. 36, 1359.

Baron, J.C., Martinot, J.L., Cambon, H., Boulenger, J.P., Poirier, M.F., Caillard, V., Blin, J., Huret, J.D., Loc'h, C., and Mazière, B. (1989) 'Striatal dopamine receptor occupancy during and following withdrawel from neuroleptic treatment: correlative evaluation by positron emission tomography and plasma prolactin levels', Psychopharmacology 99, 463.

Block, D., Coenen, H.H., Laufer, P., and Stöcklin, G. (1986) 'N.c.a. (^{18}F)-fluoroalkylation via nucleophilic fluorination of disubstituted alkanes and application to the preparation of N-(^{18}F)-fluoroethylspiperone', J. Label. Comp. Radiopharm. 23, 1042.

Block, D., Coenen, H.H., and Stöcklin, G. (1987) 'The n.c.a. nucleophilic ^{18}F-fluorination of 1,n-disubstituted alkanes as fluoroalkylation agents', J. Label. Comp. Radiopharm. 24, 1029.

Chi, D.Y., Kilbourn, M.R., Katzenellenbogen, J.A., Brodack, J.W., and Welch, M.J. (1986) 'Synthesis of no-carrier-added N-([^{18}F]fluoralkyl)spiperone derivatives', Appl. Radiat. Isot. 37,1173.

Chugani, D.C., Ackermann, R.F., and Phelps, M.E. (1988) 'In vivo [^{3}H]-spiperone binding: evidence for accumulation in corpus striatum by agonist-mediated receptor internalization', J. Cereb. Blood Flow Metab. 8, 291.

Coenen, H.H., Moerlein, S.M., and Stöcklin, G. (1983) 'No-carrier-added radiohalogenation methods with heavy halogens', Radiochimica Acta 34, 47.

Coenen, H.H., Laufer, P., Stöcklin, G., Wienhard, K., Pawlik, G., Böcher-Schwarz, H.G., and Heiss, W.-D. (1987a) '3-N-82-[^{18}F]-fluoroethyl)spiperone: A new ligand for cerebral dopamine receptor studies with PET', Life Sci. 40, 81.

Coenen, H.H., Stöcklin, G., and Wienhard, K. (1987b) 'unpublished results'.

Coenen, H.H., Wienhard, K., Stöcklin, G., Laufer, P., Heboldt, I., Pawlik, G., and Heiss, W.-D. (1988b) 'PET measurement of D_2 and S_2 receptor binding of 3-N-([2'-^{18}F]-fluoroethyl)spiperone in baboon brain', Eur. J. Nucl. Med. 14, 80.

Coenen, H.H. (1989) 'No-carrier-added ^{18}F chemistry of radiopharmaceuticals, in T.A. Baillie and J.R. Jones (eds.), Synthesis and Applications of Isotopically Labelled Compounds, Elsevier Publisher, Amsterdam, pp. 443.

Crawley, J.C., Smith, T., Veall, N., and Zanelli, G.D. (1984) 'Distribution, retention and radiation dosimetry of ^{77}Br-p-bromospiperone', Radiat. Protect. Dosimetry 8, 147-153.

Dannals, R.F., Ravert, H.T., Wilson, A.A., and Wagner Jr., H.N. (1986) 'An improved synthesis of (3-N[^{11}C]methyl)spiperone', Appl. Radiat. Isot. 37, 433.

DeJesus, O.T., Friedman, A.M., Prasad, A., and Ravenaugh, J.R. (1983) 'Preparation and purification of ^{77}Br-labelled p-bromospiroperidol suitable for in vivo dopamine receptor studies', J. Label. Comp. Radiopharm. 20, 745.

Fowler, J.S., Arnett, C.D., Wolf, A.P., Shiue, D.-Y., MacGregor, R.R., Halldin, C., Långström, B., and Wagner Jr., H.N. (1986) 'A direct comparison of the brain uptake and plasma clearance of N-[^{11}C]methylspiroperidol and [^{18}F]N-methylspiroperidol in baboon using PET', Nucl. Med. Biol. 13, 281.

Friedman, A.M., Huang, C.C., Kulmala, H.A., Dinerstein, R., Navone, J., Brundsen, B., Gawlas, D., and Cooper, M. (1982) 'The use of radiobrominated p-bromospiroperidol for gamma-ray imaging of dopamine receptors', Int. J. Nucl. Med. Biol. 9, 57-61.

Gysemans, M. and Mertens, J. (1990) 'Mechanistic approach of the nucleophilic ^{18}F-exchange on 4'-NO_2-spiperone using TBA ^{18}F or K [2.2.2.]/$^{18}F^-$', J. Label. Comp. Radiopharm. 28, 73.

Hamacher, K., Coenen, H.H., and Stöcklin, G. (1986) 'N.c.a. radiofluorination of spiperone and N-methylspiperone via aminopolyether supported direct nucleophilic substitution', J. Label. Comp. Radiopharm. 23, 1047.

Hamacher, K., Nebeling, B., Coenen, H.H., and Stöcklin, G. (1991) '[^{18}F]N-methyl-spiperone: Direct nucleophilic [^{18}F]fluorination of N-methyl-4-nitrospiperone for remote controlled routine production of n.c.a. [^{18}F]MSP', J. Label. Comp. Radiopharm. in press.

Hamacher, K., Nebeling, B., Coenen, H.H., and Stöcklin, G. (1991), to be published.

Herzog, H., Coenen, H.H., Kuwert, T., Langen, K.J., and Feinendegen, L.E. (1990) 'Quantification of the whole-body distribution of PET radiopharmaceuticals applied to 3-N-[^{18}F]fluoroethylspiperone', Eur. J. Nucl. Med. 16, 77.

Janssen, P.A.J. (1973) 'Structure-activity relationship (SAR) and drug design as illustrated with neuroleptic agents', in C.J. Cavallito (ed.), International Encyclopedia of Pharmacology and Therapeutics, Pergamon Press, Oxford, pp. 37-73.

Loc'h, C., Mazière, B., Stulzaft, O., Ottaviani, M., and Syrota, A. (1989a) 'Radioligand cerebral regional metabolism and in vivo determination of binding parameters', J. Nucl. Med. 30, 898.

Loc'h, C. and Mazière, B. (1989b) 'N.c.a. synthesis of radiohalogenated derivatives of lisuride', J. Label. Comp. Radiopharm. 26, 100.

Martinot, J.L., Paillière-Martinot, Loc'h, C., Peron Magnan, P., Mazoyer, B., Lecrubier, Y., Hardy, P., Beaufles, B., Allilaire, J.F., Mazière, B., Slama, M.F., and Syrota, A. (1990) 'Central D_2 receptors blockade and antipsychotic effects of neuroleptics', Psychiatr. and Psychobiol. 5, in press.

Mazière, B., Loc'h, C., Hantraye, P., Guillon, R., Duquesnoy, N., Soussaline, F., Naquet, R., Comar, D., and Mazière, M. (1984) '^{76}Br-bromospiroperidol: A new tool for quantitative in vivo imaging of neuroleptic receptors', Life Sci. 35, 1349.

Mazière, B. and Loc'h, C. (1986a) 'Radiopharmaceuticals labelled with bromine isotopes', Appl. Radiat. Isot. 37, 703.

Mazière, B., Loc'h, C., Stulzaft, O., Hantraye, P., Ottaviani, M., Comar, D., Mazière, M. (1986b) '^{76}Br-bromolisuride: A new tool for quantitative in vivo imaging of D_2 dopamine receptors', Eur. J. Pharmacol. 127, 239.

Mazière, B., Loc'h, C., Hantraye, P., Stulzaft, O., Martinot, J.L., Syrota, A., Mazière, M. (1990) in Bunney, Hippius, Laakmann, Schmauß, eds., Neuropsychopharmacology, Springer Verlag, pp. 409-417.

Miyazaki, H., Matsunaga, Y., Nambu, K., Oh-e, Y., Yoshida, K., and Hashimoto, M. (1986) 'Disposition and metabolism of [^{14}C]haloperidol in rats', Arzneim. Forsch./Drug Research 192, 291.

Moerlein, S.M. and Stöcklin, G. (1984) 'Radiosynthesis of n.c.a. ^{75,77}Br-bromperidol', J. Label. Comp. Radiopharm. 21, 875.

Moerlein, S.M. and Stöcklin, G. (1985) 'Synthesis of high specific activity [^{75}Br] and [^{77}Br]bromperidol and tissue distribution studies in the rat', J. Med. Chem. 28, 1319.

Moerlein, S.M., Laufer, P., Stöcklin, G., Pawlik, G., Wienhard, K., and Heiss, W.-D. (1986) 'Evaluation of ^{75}Br-labelled butyrophenone neuroleptics for imaging cerebral dopaminergic receptor areas using positron emission tomography', Eur. J. Nucl. Med. 12, 211.

Moerlein, S.M., Beyer, W., and Stöcklin, G. (1988) 'No-carrier-added radiobromination and radioiodination of aromatic rings using in situ generated peracetic acid', J. Chem. Soc., Perkin. Trans. I, 779.

Qaim, S.M. (1986) 'Recent development in the production of ^{18}F, ^{75,76,77}Br and ^{123}I', Appl. Radiat. Isot. 37, 803.

Saji, H., Nakatsuka, I., Shiba, K., Tokui, T., Horiuchi, K., Yoshitake, A., Torizuka, K., and Yokoyama, A. (1987) 'Radioiodinated 2'-iodospiperone: A new radiologand for in vivo dopamine receptor study', Life Sci. 41, 1999.

Satyamurthy, N., Bida, G., Barrio, J.R., Luxen, A., Mazziotta, J.C., Huang, S.C., and Phelps, M.E. (1986) 'No-carrier-added 3(2'-[^{18}F]fluoroethyl)spiperone, a new dopamine receptor-binding tracer for positron emission tomography', Nucl. Med. Biol. 13, 617.

Schlyer, D.J., Volkow, N.D., Fowler, J.S., Wolf, A.P., Shiue, C.-Y., Dewey, S.L., Bendrien, B., Logan, J., Raulli, R., Hitzemann, R., Brodie, J., Alavi, A.A., and McGregor, R.R. (1991) 'Regional distribution and kinetics of haloperidol binding in human brain' Arch. Gen. Psychiatry, in press.

Shiue, C.-Y., Fowler, J.S., Wolf, A.P., Watanabe, M., and Arnett, C.D. (1985) 'Synthesis and specific activity determinations of no-carrier-added (n.c.a.) fluorine-18 labeled butyrophenone neuroleptics - benperidol, haloperidol, spiroperidol, and pipamperone', J. Nucl. Med. 26, 181.

Shiue, C.-Y., Bai, L.-Q., Teng, R.-R., and Wolf, A.P. (1987) 'Syntheses of no-carrier-added (n.c.a.) [^{18}F]fluoralkylhalides and their application in the syntheses of [^{18}F]fluoroalkyl derivatives of neurotransmitter receptor active compounds' J. Label. Comp. Radiopharm. 24, 55.

Smith, M., Wolf, A.P., Brodie, J.P., Arnett, C.D., Barouche, F., Shiue, C.-Y., Fowler, J.S., Russel, J.A.G., McGregor, R.R., Wolkin, A., Angrist, B., Rottrosen, J., and Peselow, E. (1988) 'Serial [^{18}F]N-methylspiroperidol PET studies to measure changes in antipsychotic drug D_2 receptor occupancy in schizophrenic patients', Biol. Psychiatry 23, 653.

Soudijn, W., Van Wijngaarden, I., and Allewijn, F. (1967) 'Distribution excretion and metabolism of neuroleptics of the butyrophenone type. I. Excretion and metabolism of haloperidol and nine related butyrophenone-derivatives in the Wistar rat', Europ. J. Pharmacol. 1, 47-57.

Suehiro, M., Dannals, R.F., Scheffel, U., Stathis, M., Wilson, A.A., Ravert, H.T., Villemagne, V.L., Sanchez-Rao, P.M., and Wagner, H.N.J. (1990) 'In vivo labeling of the dopamine D_2 receptor with N-^{11}C-methyl-benperidol', J. Nucl. Med. 31, 2015.

Tewson, T.J., Raichle, M.E., and Welch, M.J. (1980) 'Preliminary studies with [^{18}F]haloperidol: A radioligand for in vivo studies of the dopamine receptors', Brain Res. 192, 291.

Wachtel, H., Kehr, W., and Sauer, G. (1983) 'Central antidopaminergic properties of 2-bromolisuride, an analog of the ergot dopamine agonist lisuride', Life Sci. 33, 2583.

Wagner, H.N., Burns, H.D., Dannals, R.F., Wong, D.F., Långström, B., Duelfer, T., Frost, J.J., Ravert, H.T., Links, J.M., Rosenbloom, S.B., Lukas, S.E., Kramer, A.V., and Kuhar, M.J. (1983) 'Imaging dopamine receptors in the human brain by positron tomography', Science 221, 1264.

Weissmann, A.D., Su, T.-P., Hedreen, J.C., and London, E.D. (1988) 'Sigma receptors in post-mortem human brains' J. Pharmacol. Ext. Therapeutics 247, 247.

Welch, M.J., Kilbourn, M.R., Mathias, C.J., Mintun, M.A., and Raichle, M.E. (1983) 'Comparison in animal models of ^{18}F-spiroperidol and ^{18}F-haloperidol: Potential agents for imgaging the dopamine receptor', Life Sci. 33, 1687.

Welch, M.J., Katzenellenbogen, J.A., Mathias, C.J., Brodack, J.W., Carlson, K.E., Chi, D.Y., Dence, C.S., Kilbourn, M.R., Perlmutter, J.S., Raichle, M.E., and Ter-Pogossian, M.M. (1988) 'N-(3-[^{18}F]fluoropropyl)-spiperone: The preferred ^{18}F labeled spiperone analog for positron emission tomography studies of the dopamine receptor' Nucl. Med. Biol. 15, 83.

Wienhard, K., Coenen, H.H., Pawlik, G., Rudolf, J., Laufer, P., Jovakar, S., Stöcklin, G., and Heiss, W.-D. (1990) 'PET studies of dopamine receptor distribution using [^{18}F]fluoroethylspiperone: Findings in disorders related to the dopaminergic system' J. Neuronal. Transm. 81, 195.

Wolkin, A., Brodie, J.D., Barouche, F., Rotroson, J., Wolf, A.P., Smith, M., Fowler, J.S., and Cooper, T.B. (1989) 'Dopamine receptor occupancy and plasma haloperidol levels', Arch. Gen. Psychiatry 46, 482.

RADIOLIGANDS FOR DOPAMINE RECEPTOR PET STUDIES: BENZAMIDES AND LIGANDS FOR DOPAMINE D-1 RECEPTORS

C. HALLDIN

ABSTRACT. Receptors for the endogenous neurotransmitter dopamine exist in at least two distinct subtypes, the dopamine D-1 and the D-2 receptors. Several substituted benzamides bind with high affinity and selectivity to dopamine D-2 receptors. One of them, the salicylamide [^{11}C]raclopride, has been used extensively for the *in vivo* characterization of binding to central dopamine D-2 receptors. In addition, several main types of benzamide derivatives with different side chains and/or aromatic substituents have been synthesized. The benzazepine SCH 23390 has been described as a potent dopamine D-1 receptor antagonist and [^{11}C]SCH 23390 has been used as a ligand for PET-analysis of central dopamine D-1 receptor binding in man. The benzonaphthazepine SCH 39166 has recently been characterized both *in vitro* and *in vivo* and been demonstrated to be a more selective dopamine D-1 antagonist. ^{11}C- and ^{18}F-labelled benzamides and dopamine D-1 receptor ligands for PET are reviewed.

Benzamides

STRUCTURAL CONSIDERATIONS

Substituted benzamides and butyrophenones have been the most widely used ligands for the study of dopamine D-2 receptors in the living human brain by positron emission tomography (PET) (Wagner et al., 1983; Farde *et al.*, 1986; Sedvall *et al.*, 1986a). The substituted benzamides are a recently developed class of compounds, which preferentially block the dopamine D-2 receptors (Hall *et al.*, 1988). The blockade of dopamine D-2 receptors has been shown to be closely associated with the antipsychotic effect (Seeman *et al.*, 1976; Farde *et al.*, 1988b).

There exist several main type of benzamide derivatives with different side chains and/or aromatic substituents. One common part is the 2-methoxybenzamide part often referred to as the orthopramide. The four principal types of side-chains are the following: 2-pyrrodinylmethyl (sulpiride), 4-piperidyl (clebopride), 3-pyrrolidinyl (YM 09151-2) and aminomethyl (metoclopramide). Recently, a series of compunds containing 6-methoxy (remoxipride) or 6-hydroxy (raclopride, eticlopride) substituents have been reported (de Paulis *et al.*, 1985, 1986; Hall *et al.*, 1988; Högberg *et al.*, 1990a) (Table 1).

The binding properties *in vitro* and *in vivo* of the benzamides are related to the different molecular structures. In this respect parameters such as affinity, conformation, pK_a, lipophilicity and ligand metabolism must be considered. The conformation of the salicylamides is constrained.

J. C. Baron et al. (eds.), Brain Dopaminergic Systems: Imaging with Positron Tomography, 23–38.

There is one intramolecular hydrogen bond (OH to CO) in addition to that one common for all 2-methoxybenzamides or orthopramides (NH to OMe) (Högberg *et al.*, 1986, 1987a,b). Using the stereoselective dopamine D-2 antagonist piquindone as a rigid template in molecular modelling of solid state (Högberg *et al.*, 1986) and molecular mechanics derived conformations (Högberg *et al.*, 1987a,b) the salicylamides have been suggested to have a folded of half-folded receptor-bound side chain conformation.

TABLE 1. Structural formulas of remoxipride, raclopride and eticlopride

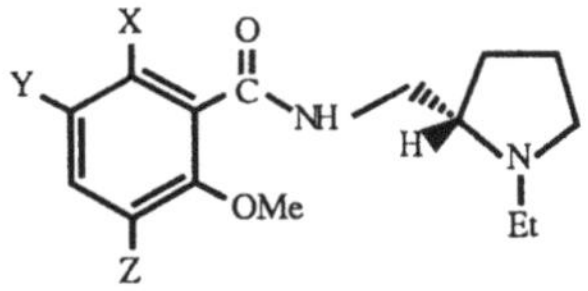

Name	X	Y	Z
remoxipride	OCH_3	Br	H
raclopride	OH	Cl	Cl
eticlopride	OH	CH_2CH_3	Cl

TABLE 2. Inhibition of [^{3}H]spiperone (IC_{50}, nM) and [^{3}H]raclopride (K_i, nM)

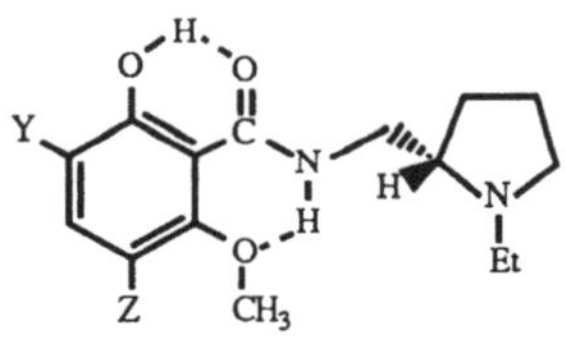

Name	Y	Z	spiperone	raclopride
raclopride	Cl	Cl	32	1.30
eticlopride	C_2H_5	Cl	0.92	0.12
FLA 797	Br	H	12	0.55
	H	OCH_3	8.8	0.75
	Cl	OCH_3	1.7	0.087
FLB 463	Br	OCH_3	1.4	0.064
NCQ 298	I	OCH_3	0.29	0.015
	C_2H_5	OCH_3	0.77	0.033
	C_3H_7	OCH_3	2.4	0.023

A number of salicylamide analogues are shown in Table 2 (Högberg *et al.*, 1990a). The affinity of the different analogues was measured by inhibition of [^{3}H]spiperone (IC_{50}, nM) and [^{3}H]raclopride (K_i, nM) binding. The replacement of the 3-chloro group (Y) in raclopride with the 3-ethyl group in eticlopride leads to a 30-fold higher affinity. One of the most potent and selective compounds shown is the iodo derivate NCQ 298 which inhibites the [^{3}H]spiperone binding by 0.29 nM (IC_{50}) and [^{3}H]raclopride binding by 0.015 nM (K_i). This makes NCQ 298 suitable as a radioligand (in the ^{123}I-labelled form) for SPECT (Högberg *et al* ., 1990c; Hall *et al.*, 1991a).

Benzamides with a N-ethyl side chain display the (S)-enantiomer as the more potent antipode. However, the corresponding substituted N-benzyl derivatives have the affinity confined to the (R)-enatiomer as shown in Table 3. Inhibition of [^{3}H]spiperone binding gave an affinity of 0.65 and 126 nM (IC_{50}) for the (R)- and (S)-enantiomers, respectively (Högberg *et al* ., 1991a,b).

Many 5-substituted 2,3-dimethoxybenzamides display a remarkably high affinity for the dopamine D-2 site (Högberg *et al* ., 1990b,d) (Table 4). The electronic influence of the 5-substituent (Y) seem to be of minor imortance which is also in line with the behaviour of the corresponding salicylamides. These characteristics makes the alkyl derivatives (for example No 6 and 7) suitable also for ^{18}F-labelling (Mathis *et al.*, 1990; Mukherjee *et al.*, 1990).

TABLE 3. Inhibition of [^{3}H]spiperone binding (IC_{50}, nM)

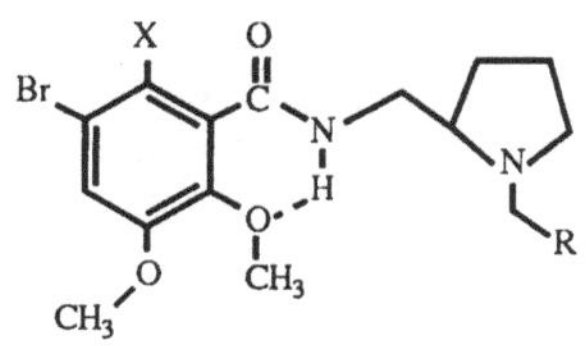

R	Sterochem.	X=OH	X=H
CH_3	S	1.4 (FLB 463)	1.2 (FLB 457)
CH_3	R	79	145
$CH{=}CH_2$	S	2.3	1.5
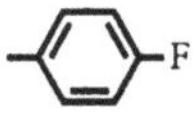	S	--	126
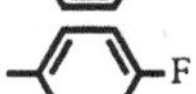	R	1.3 (NCQ 117)	0.65 (NCQ 115)

TABLE 4. Inhibition of [^{3}H]spiperone binding

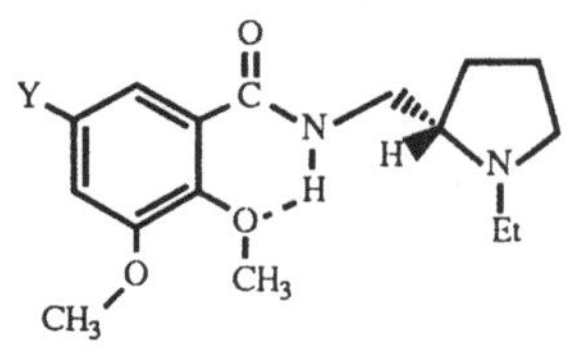

No	Y	IC_{50}, nM
1	H	52
2	Cl	0.4
3	Br	1.2
4	I	0.7
5	CH_3	5.2
6	C_2H_5	1.3
7	C_4H_9	2.7
8	SCH_3	1.1
9	$Si(CH_3)_3$	3.5

[^{11}C]Raclopride

The research on the biological role of dopamine D-2 receptors has been stimulated by the availabilty of several D-2-selective compounds. Raclopride ((-)-(S)-3,5-dichloro-N-((1-ethyl-2-pyrrolidinyl)methyl)-6-methoxysalicylamide) has in animal experiments been shown to be a potent and selective antagonist of dopamine D-2 receptors. (Köhler *et al.*, 1985; Hall *et al.*, 1988). *In vitro* studies showed that [^{3}H]raclopride binds with high affinity (K_d = 1.2 nM and a low proportion of non-specific binding to rat striatal homogenates. The binding of [^{3}H]raclopride is saturable (B_{max} = 23.5 pmol/g wet wt) and reversible (dissociation half life = 30 min). After *in vivo* administration, [^{3}H]raclopride accumulates preferentially in dopamine rich brain areas with approximately 10 times higer levels in the striatum than in the cerebellum . The *in vivo* binding was saturable, reversible and showed a low non.specific binding. More than 90 % of the radioactivity retained in the brain after 45 minutes represented unchanged [^{3}H]raclopride.

[^{11}C]Raclopride has been labelled with ^{11}C either by N-ethylation with [^{11}C]ethyl iodide (Ehrin *et al.*, 1985) or by O-methylation with [^{11}C]methyl iodide (Farde *et al.*, 1988a; Halldin *et al.*, 1991) (Scheme 1). Both [^{11}C]methyl iodide and [^{11}C]ethyl iodide can be routinely prepared from [^{11}C]carbon dioxide. When using [^{11}C]ethyl iodide, longer reaction time and lower specific radioactivity are obtained compared to [^{11}C]methyl iodide. These factors make O-methylation more suitable for routine synthesis than N-ethylation.

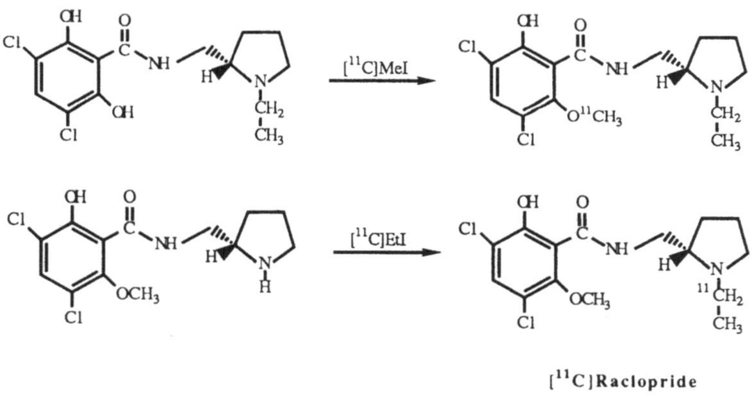

Scheme 1.

[^{11}C]Raclopride has been used for: a) saturation studies to determine B_{max} and K_d in neuroleptic-naive schizophrenic patients (Farde *et al.*, 1986, 1990) b) receptor occupancy studies of schizophrenic patients treated with antipsychotic drugs (Farde *et al.*, 1988b) c) stereoselectivity-studies of raclopride using both + and - enantiomers (Farde *et al.*, 1988a) d) development of a kinetic analytical model in comparison to the equilibrium model (Farde *et al.*, 1989a) e) dopamine D-2 receptor determination in pituitary adenomas (Muhr *et al.*, 1988) and f) receptor supersensitivity studies in patients with Parkinsons disease (Rinne *et al.*, 1990).

[^{11}C]Eticlopride

Eticlopride is a substituted salicylamide with a 30-fold higher affinity for dopamine D-2 receptors than raclopride (Table 2). The compound is highly selective since the affinity for other putative central receptors are negligible. Eticlopride has been labelled with ^{11}C in two different positions; in the N-ethyl group and in the O-methyl group (Halldin *et al.*, 1990b). The strategy of labelling eticlopride with ^{11}C in the N-ethyl group by using [^{11}C]ethyl iodide was similar to the method used for [N-ethyl-^{11}C]raclopride.

The synthesis of [O-methyl-^{11}C]eticlopride was more complicated because, unlike the diphenolic precursor used for the synthesis of [O-methyl-^{11}C]raclopride (Scheme 1) the required diphenol is unsymmetrical in the present precursor molecule (Scheme 2). The methylation was followed by a HPLC-separation of the two different O-methylated products. This method has the advantage of using [^{11}C]methyl iodide instead of [^{11}C]ethyl iodide (e.g. higher specific radioactivity).

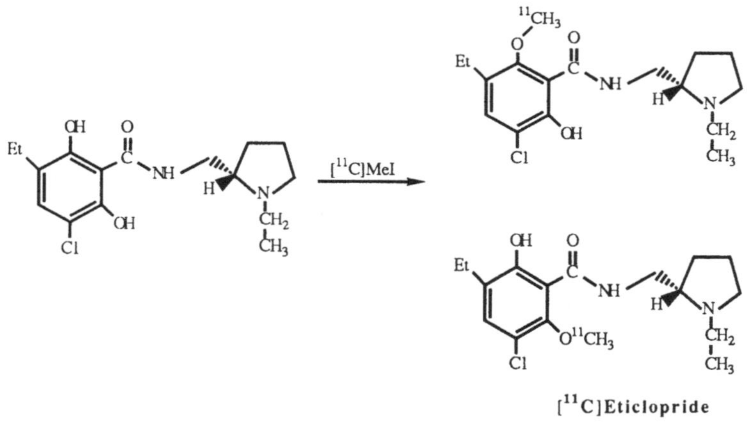

Scheme 2.

After i.v. injection of [^{11}C]eticlopride into a cynomolgus monkey the ratio of radioactivity in the striatum to cerebellum increased linearily with time and was about 2.5 after 57 minutes (no.II, Figure 1). This linear increase implied that a kinetic analysis should be more appropriate than an equilibrium analysis (cf spiperone analogs). The high selectivity may together with the high affinity allow examination of dopamine D-2 receptors in extrastriatal regions in the human brain by PET (Halldin *et al.*, 1990b; Halldin *et al.*, 1991).

Other [^{11}C]-labelled benzamides

FLB 524 is another benzamide that has been labelled with ^{11}C and used in PET (Farde *et al.*, 1985). However, this ligand has too low affinity and too high non-specific binding to be a valuable tool for the study of dopamine D-2 receptors.

The commercial drug remoxipride (Roxiam, Astra) has also been labelled with ^{11}C (Farde *et al.*, 1989b). The compound passed the blood-brain-barrier but showed no specific binding. This low specific binding is expected because of the low affinity of remoxipride for dopamine D-2 receptors (200 nM).

[^{11}C]YM-09151-2 has been prepared and so far reported only after studies in rats and dogs (Hatano *et al.*, 1989). This compound has a higher affinity for dopamine D-2 receptors than that of raclopride. The potantiel of the compound as a PET-ligand for human studies has not yet been evaluated.

[^{11}C]Clebopride has been prepared (Guan *et al.*, 1989) only with a low specific activity of 0.2 Ci/mmol. The potential of the ligand for labelling dopamine D-2 receptors is therefore uncertain.

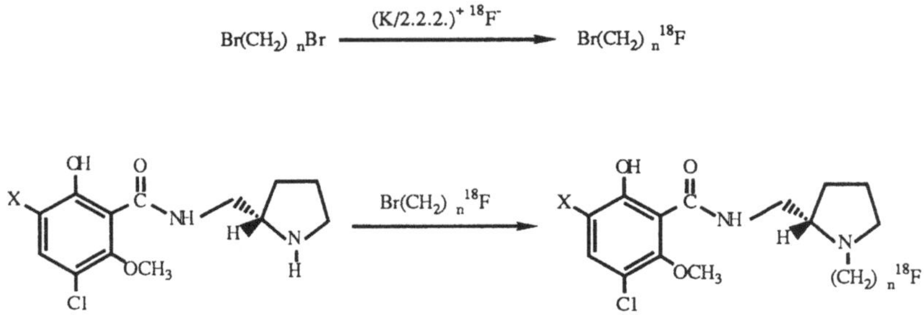

Compound	X	n
NCQ 258	Cl	2
NCQ 134	CH_3CH_2	2
NCQ 135	CH_3CH_2	3

Scheme 3.

[^{18}F]-Labelled raclopride, eticlopride and YM-09151-2 analogues

Several spiperone derivatives labelled with positron-emitting isotopes have higher affinity for the dopamine D-2 receptors and also higher striatum to cerebellum ratios than [^{11}C]raclopride. High ratios are in particular demonstrated at late times after injection of ^{18}F-labelled spiperone derivatives. However, a severe problem with the spiperone derivatives used so far is a considerable affinity to $5HT_2$-receptors.

To allow the study of ligand distribution for a longer time with PET a raclopride analogue labelled with fluorine-18 in the β-position of the N-ethyl group, [^{18}F]NCQ 258 (III), has been prepared by several groups (Halldin *et al.*, 1988, 1989a, 1989b, 1991; Kiesewetter *et al.*, 1989, 1990; Lannoye *et al.*, 1989, 1990). However, the affinity *in vitro* was lowered 3-5 times for NCQ 258 as compared to raclopride.

A similar substitution in the N-ethyl group of the considerably more potent salicylamide eticlopride was performed (Halldin *et al.*, 1989b, 1991; Lannoye *et al.*, 1990). To reduce the inductive influence on the pyrrolidine nitrogen the γ-fluorinated N-propyl analog was also prepared. [^{18}F]NCQ 258 (**III**), [^{18}F]NCQ 134 (**IV**) and [^{18}F]NCQ 135 (**V**) were prepared from [^{18}F]-2-fluoroethyl bromide and [^{18}F]-3-fluoropropyl bromide, respectively (Halldin *et al.*, 1991) (Scheme 3).

[^{11}C]raclopride, [^{11}C]eticlopride and compounds **III-V** were injected into cynomolgus monkeys for PET-examination of ligand distribution in brain *in vivo* (Halldin *et al.*, 1991) (Figure 6). The PET-experiments showed that the N-ethyl group of the salicylamides, raclopride and eticlopride, should not be substituted with a β-fluoro group (**III-IV**). Of the ^{18}F-labelled salicylamides studied here the γ-fluoro analog [^{18}F]NCQ 135 (**V**) was the only one reported possible for visualization of dopamine D-2 receptors by PET.

The results indicate that it is difficult to predict the *in vivo* binding properties of analogues and that *in vitro* binding studies can not be used categorically to predict a tracer for *in vivo* PET studies. This underlines that *in vivo* conditions like protein binding, non-specific binding, temperature effects or ligand metabolism (as defluorination (Lannoye *et al.*, 1990)) may be involved.

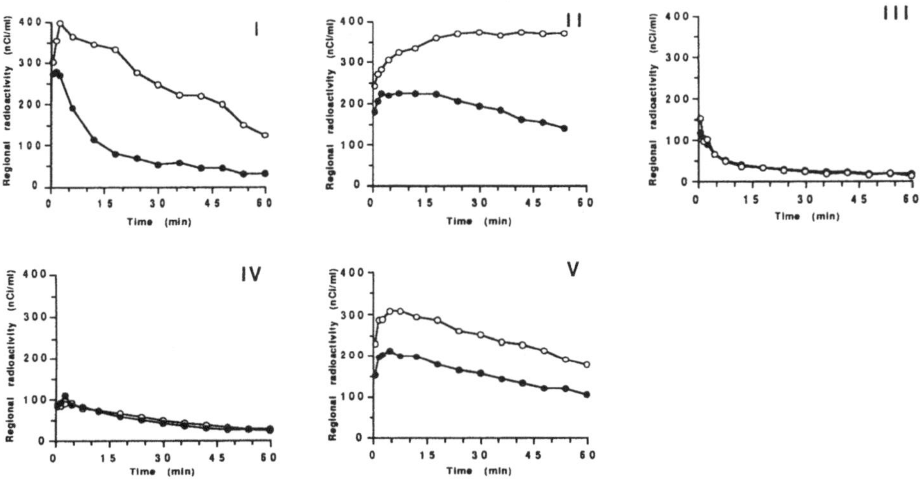

Figure 1. Regional radioactivity (nCi/mL) versus time (min) for two brain regions after i.v. injection of the compounds [^{11}C]raclopride (**I**), [^{11}C]eticlopride (**II**), [^{18}F]NCQ 258 (**III**), [^{18}F]NCQ 134 (**IV**) and [^{18}F]NCQ 135 (**V**), open circles = striatum, filled circles = cerebellum.

Two [^{18}F]fluoroalkyl analogues of YM-09151-2 have been prepared recently. The [^{18}F]fluoropropyl analogue was shown to have a striatum to cerebellum ratio, in *in vivo* rat studies, comparable to that of [^{11}C]YM-09151-2 and was concluded to be a good candidate for measuring dopamine-D-2 receptors *in vivo* (Hatano *et al.*, 1990).

[^{18}F]NCQ 115

NCQ 115 ((+)-(R)-5-bromo-N-((1-(4-fluorobenzyl)-2-pyrrolidinyl)-methyl)-2,3-dimethoxybenzamide) is a selective D-2 dopamine receptor antagonist. The compound inhibits potently the binding of [^{3}H]raclopride (K_i = 147 pM) and has an F in the benzyl group (Hall *et al.*, 1991b).[^{18}F]NCQ 115 was therefore suggested as a potential ^{18}F-labelled benzamide for PET (Halldin *et al.*, 1990c).

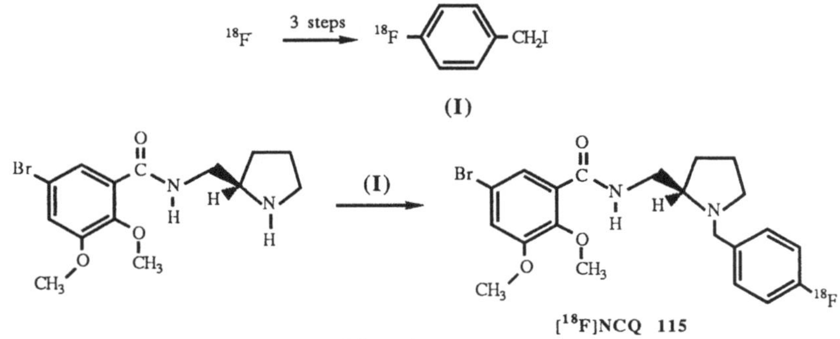

Scheme 4.

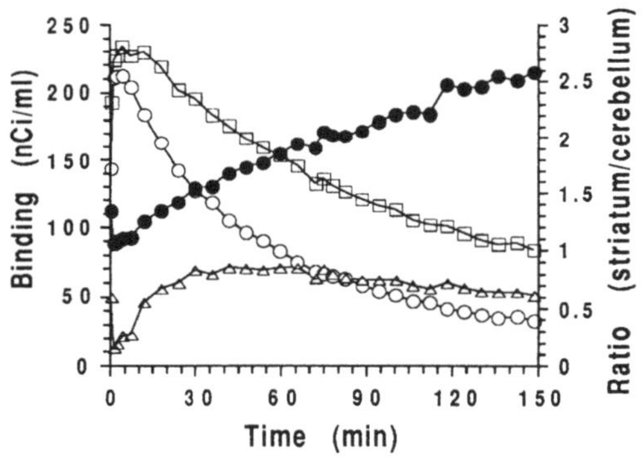

Figure 2. Time course of radioactivity in striatum (squares) and cerebellum (open circles) in a Cynomolgus monkey after administration of 45 MBq [^{18}F]NCQ 115. Shown is also specific binding, defined as radioactivity in the striatum minus that in the cerebellum (triangles) and ratio of radioactivity striatum/cerebellum (filled circles).

[^{18}F]NCQ 115 was prepared from [^{18}F]fluoride ion via [^{18}F]-4-fluorobenzyl iodide (Scheme 4). For binding studies *in vitro* ^{3}H-labelled NCQ 115 was also prepared. Binding with high affinity and high selectivity to dopamine D-2 receptors in both rat striatum and in human caudate was demonstrated. [^{18}F]NCQ 115 was used in PET visualization of the dopamine receptor rich areas of the monkey brain (Halldin *et al.*, 1990b). The results shows a conspicuous uptake of radioactivity in the monkey striatum and a possible equilibrium after 60-90 min (Figure 2). [^{18}F]NCQ 115 was concluded to be a possible PET ligand for D-2 dopamine receptors in man.

5-[^{18}F]Fluoroalkylbenzamides

The remarkably high affinity for the dopamine D-2 site by the 5-substituted 2,3-dimethoxybenzamides is shown in Table 4. There is only a minor influence of the 5-substituent. A series of 2,3-dimethoxy-5-fluoroalkylbenzamides have been synthesized (Mathis *et al.*, 1990) (Table 5). Compounds 2-5 have also been labelled with ^{18}F. Striatum to cerebellum radioactivity ratios following injection of ^{18}F-3 and ^{18}F-5 in rats was reported to increase steadily to >100/1 at 5h (Mathis *et al.*, 1990). Preliminary PET-studies in Cebus apella using ^{18}F-3 show localization of the radiotracer in the striatum with the ratio of striatum to cerebellum increasing from 1.38 at 16 min to 3.05 at 120 min (Mukherjee *et al.*, 1990). These results indicates the potential of these compounds as ligands for dopamine D-2 studies using PET.

TABLE 5. Aryl-substituted (S)-N-((1-ethyl-2-pyrrolidinyl)-methyl)-2,3-dimethoxy-5-(fluoroalkyl)benzamides

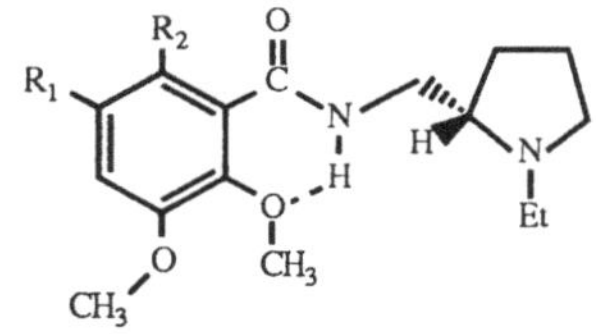

No	R1	R2
1	I	H
2	CH_2CH_2F	H
3	$CH_2CH_2CH_2F$	H
4	CH_2CH_2F	OH
5	$CH_2CH_2CH_2F$	OH
6	$CH_2CH_2CH_2OTs$	H
7	$CH_2CH_2CH_2OTs$	OMEM
8	$CH_2CH_2CH_2F$	OMEM

Ligands For Dopamine D-1 Receptors

INTRODUCTION

The examination of central dopamine D-1 receptor characteristics and function has been hampered because of the previous lack of selective dopamine D-1 receptor compounds. A few years ago the benzazepine SCH 23390 ((R)-(+)-8-chloro-2,3,4,5-tetrahydro-3-methyl-5-phenyl-1H-3-benzazepin-7-ol) was described as a potent dopamine D-1 receptor antagonist with an, compared to classical neuroleptics, atypical pharmacological profile (Iorio, 1981; Hyttel, 1983). $[^3H]$SCH 23390 was shown to bind selectively to D-1 receptors in membanes of the rat and human striatum (Billard *et al.*, 1984; Raisman *et al.*, 1985; Schultz *et al.*, 1985; Pimoule *et al.*, 1985). In animal experiments the dopamine D-1 receptors mediate behavioural effects (for review see Waddington and O'Boyle, 1989). The pharmacological effect of a selective D-1 antagonist on schizophrenic patients has not yet been examined. PET studies with the radiobrominated analogue $[^{76}Br]$SCH 23390 indicated that the analog accumulated in the striatum of the monkey brain (Friedman *et al.*, 1985). The $[^{18}F]$fluoroethyl analogue of SCH 23390 has also been prepared (Moerlein *et al.*, 1989). The potential of this fluoroethyl-analog of SCH 23390 as PET-ligand has not yet been clarified. It is known that by substitution of the N-methyl with a N-ethyl decreases the affinity by about two orders of magnitude (K_d = 0.4 nM compared to 41 nM).

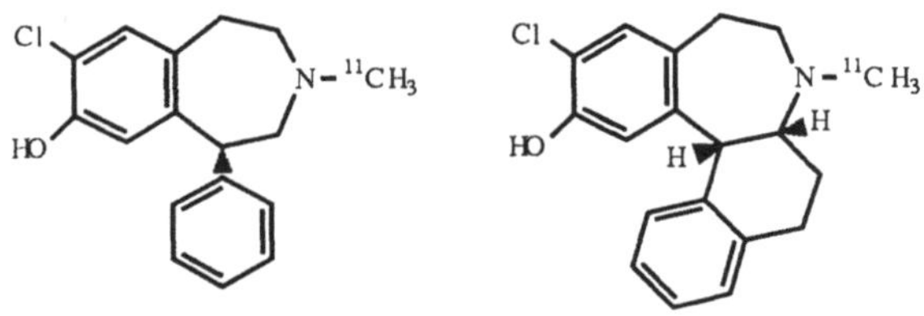

$[^{11}C]$SCH 23390 $[^{11}C]$SCH 39166

Figure 3. Structural formulas of $[^{11}C]$SCH 23390 and $[^{11}C]$SCH 39166

RADIOLIGANDS

$[^{11}C]$SCH 23390

$[^{11}C]$SCH 23390 has been prepared by alkylation of the desmethyl compound SCH 24518 ((R)-(+)-8-chloro-2,3,4,5-tetrahydro-5-phenyl-1H-3-benzazepin-7-ol) with $[^{11}C]$methyl iodide (Halldin *et al.*, 1986; DeJesus *et al.*, 1987; Ravert *et al.*, 1987) (Figure 3). The usefulness of $[^{11}C]$SCH 23390 as ligand for PET-analysis of central dopamine D-1 receptor binding in monkey and man is well established (Halldin *et al.*, 1986; Sedvall *et al.*, 1986b; Farde *et al.*, 1987). PET-analysis of human receptor subtypes using $[^{11}C]$SCH 23390 has been performed in healthy volunteers and drug-treated schizophrenic patients (Farde *et al.*, 1987). Age-related changes in human D-1 dopamine receptors have been measured by PET (Suhara *et al.*, 1991). Different behaviour of striatal dopamine D-1 and D-2 receptors in early Parkinson's disease have been demonstrated by PET using $[^{11}C]$SCH 23390 and $[^{11}C]$raclopride (Rinne *et al.*, 1990). However, $[^{11}C]$SCH 23990 has significant affinity also for $5HT_2$-receptors and is rapidly metabolised (80-90%) during the time of a PET-experiment (1 hour).

[^{11}C]SCH 39166

The benzonaphthazepine SCH 39166 ((-)-trans-6,7,7a,8,9,13b-hexahydro-3-chloro-2-hydroxy-N-methyl-5H-benzo(d)naphtho-(2,1-b)azepine) has recently been characterized both *in vitro* and *in vivo* and has been demonstrated to be a selective dopamine D-1 antagonist (Chipkin et al., 1988). In animals SCH 39166 is more slowly metabolized than SCH 23990. Both SCH 23390 and SCH 39166 has a nanomolar affinity for dopamine D-1 receptors. However, SCH 39166 has an about 25-fold lower affinity for $5HT_2$-receptors and is thus a more selective dopamine D-1 receptor ligand than SCH 23390. The compound is undergoing clinic trials as a potential antipsychotic drug.

In contrast to SCH 23390, SCH 39166 has 2 asymmetric carbon atoms located in a trans conformation (Figure 3). For the 4 stereoisomers the affinity to dopamine D-1 receptors has been investigated *in vitro* (Berger *et al.*, 1989). The affinity of SCH 39166 for the dopamine D-1 receptor is 300-500 times higher as compared to the affinity of the other stereoisomers.

[^{11}C]SCH 39166 was labelled by N-methylation of the free base of the secondary amine in acetone with [^{11}C]methyl iodide (Halldin *et al.*, 1990a; Adam *et al.*, 1990) (Scheme 5). [^{11}C]SCH 39166 have been examined as a potential PET-ligand (Sedvall *et al.*, 1991). [^{11}C]SCH 39166 was injected i.v. into a cynomolgus monkey . There was a rapid accumulation of radioactivity in the brain (Figure 4). PET-analysis demonstrated accumulation in the striatum, a region known to have a high density of dopamine D-1 receptors (Figure 4a). In a second experiment, radioactivity in the striatum but not in the receptor poor cerebellum was markedly reduced after injection of 6 mg unlabelled SCH 23390 (Figure 4b). In a second displacement experiment the effect of a high dose (5 mg) ketanserin was investigated. No reduction of specific binding in the striatum or neocortex was demonstrated. This displacement experiments indicates the specificity and reversibility of [^{11}C]SCH 39166 binding to dopamine D-1 receptors. [^{11}C]SCH 39166 was concluded to be a possible PET ligand for dopamine D-1 receptors in man (Sedvall *et al.*, 1991).

Scheme 5.

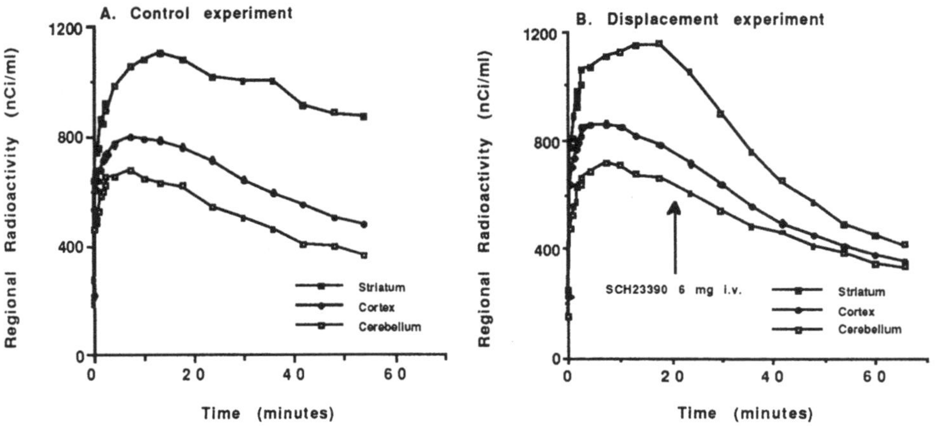

Figure 4. Regional radioactivity (nCi/mL) vs time (min) in the brain of a Cynomolgus monkey after i.v. administration of 40 MBq of [^{11}C]SCH 39166. (A) Control experiment; (B) displacement experiment.

Acknowledgements. I am grateful to all my coauthors in the cited references and I will especially thank Lars Farde, Håkan Hall, Thomas Högberg and Göran Sedvall for a fruitful collaboration. Substantial support was granted from the National Institute of Mental Health (NIMH, Grant No. 5664710-0)

References

Adam M.J., Duelfer T. and Ruth T.J. (1990) Synthesis of C-11 labelled SCH 39166 a potential D1 dopamine antagonist for PET studies. *J. Nucl. Med.* **31**, 737.

Berger J.G., Chang W.K., Clader J.W., Hou D., Chipkin R.E. and McPhail A.T. (1989) Synthesis and receptor affinities of some conformationally restricted analogues of the dopamine D_1 selective ligand (5R)-8-chloro-2,3,4,5-tetrahydro-3-methyl-5-phenyl-1H-3-benzazepin-7-ol *J. Med. Chem.* **32**, 1913.

Billard W., Ruperto V., Crosby G., Iorio L.C. and Barnett A. (1984) Characterization of the binding of ^{3}H-SCH 23390, a selective D-1 receptor antagonist ligand, in rat striatum. *Life. Sci.* **35**, 1885.

Chipkin R.E., Iorio L.C., Coffin V.L., Mcquade R.D., Berger J.G. and Barnett A.J. (1988) Pharmacological profile of SCH 39166: A dopamine D1 selective benzonaphtazepine with potential antipsychotic activity.*Pharmacol. Exp. Ther.* **247**,1093.

DeJesus O.T., van Moffart G.J.C. and Friedman A.M. (1987) Synthesis of [^{11}C]SCH 23390 for dopamine D1 receptor studies. (1987) *Appl. Radiat. Isot.* **38**, 345.

de Paulis T., Hall H., Ögren S-O., Wägner A., Stensland B. and Csöregh I. (1985) Synthesis, crystal structure and antidopaminergic properties of eticlopride (FLB 131). *Eur. J. Med. Chem.* **20**, 273.

de Paulis T., Kumar Y., Johansson L., Rämsby S., Hall H., Sällemark M., Ängeby-Möller K. and Ögren S-O. (1986) Potential neuroleptic agents. 4. Chemistry, behavioral pharmacology, and inhibition of [^{3}H]spiperone binding of 3,5-disubstututed N-[(1-ethyl-2-pyrrolidinyl)-methyl]-6-methoxysalicylamides. *J. Med. Chem.* **29**, 61.

Ehrin E., Farde L., de Paulis T., Eriksson L., Greitz T., Johnström P., Litton J-E., Nilsson L., Sedvall G., Stone-Elander S. and Ögren S-O. (1985) Preparation of ^{11}C-labelled raclopride, a new potent dopamine receptor anatgonist: prelininary PET studies of cerebral dopamine receptors in the monkey. *Int. J. Appl. Radiat. Isot.* **36**, 269.

Farde L., Ehrin E., Eriksson L., Greitz T.Y., Hall. H., Hedström C.G., Litton J-E. and Sedvall G. (1985) Substituted benzamides as ligands for visualization of dopamine receptor binding in the human brain by positron emission tomography. *Proc. Natl. Acad. Sci. USA* **82**, 3863.

Farde L., Hall H., Ehrin E. and Sedvall G. (1986) Quantitative analysis of dopamine D2 receptor binding in the living human brain by positron emission tomography. *Science* **231**, 258.

Farde L., Halldin C., Stone-Elander S. and Sedvall G. (1987) Analysis of human dopamine receptor subtypes using ^{11}C-SCH 23390 and ^{11}C-raclopride. *Psychopharmacology* **92**, 278.

Farde L., Pauli S., Hall H., Eriksson L., Halldin C., Högberg T., Nilsson L., Sjögren I. and Stone-Elander S. (1988a) Stereoselective binding of ^{11}C-raclopride in living human brain - a search for extrastriatal central D2-dopamine receptors by PET. *Psychopharmacology* **94**, 471.

Farde L., Wiesel F-A., Halldin C. and Sedvall G. (1988b) Central D2-dopamine receptor occupancy in schizophrenic patients treated with antipsychotic drugs. *Arch. Gen. Psychiatry* **45**, 71.

Farde L., Eriksson L., Blomquist G. and Halldin C. (1989a) Kinetic analysis of ^{11}C-raclopride binding to D2-dopamine receptors studied by PET - a comparison to the equilibrium analysis. *J. Cer. Blood Flow Met.* **9**, 696.

Farde L. and von Bahr C. (1989b) Distribution of remoxipride to the human brain and central D2-dopamine receptor binding examined in vivo by PET. *Acta Psychiatr. Scand.* **82**, 67.

Farde L., Wiesel F-A., Stone-Elander S., Halldin C., Nordström A-L., Hall H. and Sedvall G. (1990) D2-dopamine receptors in neuroleptic-naive schizophrenic patients - a PET-study with [^{11}C]raclopride. *Arch. Gen. Psychiatry.* **47**, 213.

Friedman A., DeJesus O.T., Woolverton W.L., van Moffart G., Goldberg L.T., Prasad A., Barnett A. and Dinerstein R. (1985) Positron tomography of radiobrominated analog of the D1/DA1 antagonist, SCH 23390. *Eur. J. Pharmacol.* **108**, 327.

Guan J.H., Livni E. and Elmaleh. (1989). [^{11}C]clebopride: a novel D2-antagonist as a potential D2-receptor tracer for PET. *J. Lab. Comp. Radiopharm.* **26**, 215.

Hall H., Köhler C., Gawell L., Farde L. and Sedvall G. (1988) Raclopride, a new selective ligand for the dopamine-D2 receptors. *Prog. Neuro- Psychopharmacol. and Biol. Psychiat.* **12**, 559.

Hall H., Högberg T., Halldin C., Köhler C., Ström P., Ross S.B., Larsson S.A. and Farde L. (1991) NCQ 298, a new selective iodinated salicylamide ligand for the labelling of dopamine D_2 receptors. *Psychopharmacology* **103**, 6.

Hall H., Högberg T., Halldin C., Bengtsson S. and Wedel I. (1991) Synthesis and binding properties of the fluorinated substituted benzamide [^{3}H]NCQ 115, a new selective dopamine D_2 receptor ligand. *Mol. Pharmacol.* (in press).

Halldin C., Stone-Elander S., Farde L., Ehrin E., Fasth K-J., Långström B. and Sedvall G. (1986) Preparation of ^{11}C-labelled SCH 23390 for the *in vivo* study of dopamine D-1 receptors using positron emission tomography. *Appl. Radiat. Isot.* **37**, 1039.

Halldin C., Högberg T., Stone-Elander S., Farde L., Hall H., Printz G., Solin O. and Sedvall G. (1988) Synthesis of [ethyl-^{18}F]fluororaclopride for the in vivo study of dopamine D2 receptors using PET. *J. Nucl. Med.* **29**, 767.

Halldin C., Farde L., Hall H., Högberg T., Printz G., Pulka W., Sedvall G. and Solin O. (1989a) Synthesis and PET-comparison of five benzamide analogs. Presented at The Fifth Symposium on the Medical Application of Cyclotrons, Turku, Finland, 1989. *Acta Radiol. Proc.* (In press).

Halldin C., Högberg T., Stone-Elander S., Farde L., Hall H., Printz G., Solin O. and Sedvall G. (1989b) Synthesis of [ethyl-^{18}F]fluororaclopride for the in vivo study of dopamine D2 receptors using PET. *J. Lab. Comp. Radioparm.* **26**, 338.

Halldin C., Farde L., Barnett A. and Sedvall G. (1990a) Preparation of [^{11}C]SCH 39166, a new selective D-1 dopamine receptor ligand for PET. *J. Nucl. Med.* **31**, 737.

Halldin C., Farde L., Högberg T., Hall H., and Sedvall G. (1990b) ^{11}C-Labelling of eticlopride in two different positions - a selective high-affinity ligand for the study of dopamine D-2 receptors using PET. *Appl. Radiat. Isot.* **41**, 669.

Halldin C., Högberg T., Bengtsson S., Hall H. and Farde L. (1990c) Preparation of [^{18}F]NCQ 115, a new selective reversible D-2 dopamine receptor ligand for PET. *J. Nucl. Med.* **31**, 902.

Halldin C., Farde L., Högberg T., Hall H., Ström P., Ohlberger A. and Solin O. (1991) A comparative PET-study of five carbon-11 or fluorine-18 labelled salicylamides. Preparation and in vitro dopamine D-2 receptor binding. *Nucl. Med. Biol.* (In press).

Hatano K., Ischiwata K., Kawashima K., Hatazawa J., Itoh M, and Ido T. (1989) D2-dopamine receptor specific brain uptake of carbon-11-labeled YM-09151-2. *J. Nucl. Med.* **30**, 515.

Hatano K., Ido T., Ischiwata K., Hatazawa J., Itoh M., Kawashima K. and Iwata R. (1990) Synthesis of w-[^{18}F]fluoroalkyl analogs of YM-09151-2 for the measurement of D2-dopamine receptors with PET. *Appl. Radiat. Isot.* **41**, 551.

Högberg T., Rämsby S., de Paulis T., Stensland B., Csöregh I. and Wägner A. (1986) Solid state conformations and antidopaminergic effects of remoxipride hydrochloride and a closely related salicylamide, FLA 797, in relation to dopamine receptor models. *Mol. Pharmacol.* **30**, 345.

Högberg T., Norinder U., Rämsby S. and Stensland B. (1987a) Crystallographic, theoretical and molecular modelling studies on the conformations of the salicylamide, raclopride, a selective dopamine D-2 antagonist. *J. Pharm. Pharmacol.* **39**, 787.

Högberg T., Rämsby S., Ögren S-O. and Norinder U. (1987b) New selective dopamine D-2 antagonists as antipsychotic agents, Pharmacological, chemical, structural and theoretical considerations. *Acta Pharm. Suec.* **24**, 289.

Högberg T., Bengtsson S., de Paulis T., Johansson L., Ström P., Hall H. and Ögren S.O. (1990a) Potential antipsychotic agents. 5. Synthesis and antidopaminergic properties of substituted 5,6-dimethoxysalicylamides and related compounds. A comparative study. *J. Med. Chem.* **33,** 1155.

Högberg T., de Paulis T., Johansson L., Kumar Y., Hall H. and Ögren S.O. (1990b) Potential antipsychotic agents. 7. Synthesis and antidopaminergic properties of the atypical highly potent (S)-5-bromo-2,3-dimethoxy-N-((1-ethyl-2-pyrrolidinyl)methyl)benzamide and related compounds. A comparative study. *J. Med. Chem.* **33,** 2305.

Högberg T., Ström P., Hall H., Köhler C., Halldin C. and Farde L. (1990c) Syntheses of [^{123}I]-, [^{125}I]- and unlabelled (S)-3-iodo-5,6-dimethoxy-N-((1-ethyl-2-pyrrolidinyl)methyl)salicylamide (NCQ 298), selective ligands for the study of dopamine D-2 receptors. *Acta Pharm. Nord.* **2,** 53.

Högberg T., Ström P., Hall H. and Ögren S.O. (1990d) Potential antipsychotic agents. 8. Antidopaminergic properties of a potent series of 5-substituted (-)-(S)-N-((1-ethylpyrrolidin-2-yl)methyl)-2,3-dimethoxybenzamides. Synthesis via common lithio intermediates. *Helv. Chim. Acta* **73,** 417.

Högberg T., Ström P., de Paulis T., Stensland B., Csöregh I., Lundin K., Hall H. and Ögren S.O. (1991a) Potential antipsychotic agents. 9. Synthesis and stereoselective dopamine D-2 receptor blockade of a potent class of substituted (R)-N-((1-benzyl-2-pyrrolidinyl)methyl)benzamides. Relation to other side chain congeners. *J. Med. Chem.* (in press).

Högberg T. (1991b) Novel substituted salicylamides and benzamides as selective dopamine D_2 receptor antagonists. *Drugs Fut..* (in press).

Hyttel J. (1983) SCH 23390 - the first slective dopamine D1 antagonist. *Eur. J. Pharmacol.* **91,** 153.

Iorio L.C. (1981) SCH 23390. A benzazepine with a atypical effects on dopaminergic systems. *The Pharmacologist* **23,** 136.

Kebabian J.W. and Calne D.B. (1979) Multiple receptors for dopamine. *Nature* **277,** 960.

Kiesewetter D.O., Brucke T. and Finn R.D. (1989) Radiochemical synthesis of [^{18}F]fluororaclopride. *Appl. Radiat. Isot.* **40,** 455.

Kiesewetter D.O., Kawai R., Chelliah M., Owens E., Mclellan C. and Blasberg R.G. (1990) Preparation and biological evaluation of ^{18}F-labeled analogs as potential dopamine D_2receptor ligands. *Nucl. Med. Biol.* **17,** 347.

Köhler C., Hall H., Ögren S-O. and Gawell L. (1985) Specific in vitro and in vivo binding of [^{3}H]raclopride. A potent substituted benzamide drug with high affinity for dopamine D-2 receptors in the rat brain. *Biochem. Pharmac.* **34** , 2251.

Lannoye G.S., Moerlein S.M. and Welch M.J. (1989) Radiosynthesis of N-(w-[^{18}F]fluoroalkyl) derivatives of the dopaminergic receptor-binding ligand raclopride. *J. Lab. Comp. Radiopharm.* **26,** 340.

Lannoye G.S., Moerlein S.M., Parkinson D. and Welch M.J. (1990) N-Fluoroalkylated and N-alkylated analogues of the dopaminergic D-2 receptor antagonist raclopride. *J. Med. Chem.* **33,** 2430.

Mathis C.A., Bishop J.E., Gerdes J.M., Faggin B. and Mailman R. (1990) Synthesis of aryl-substituted 5-[^{18}F]fluoroalkylbenzamides: high affinity ligands for dopamine D-2 studies. *J. Lab. Comp. Radiopharm.* (in press).

Moerlein S.M., Lannoye G.S. and Welch M.J. (1989) No-carrier-added synthesis of N-w-(F-18)fluoroethyl SCH-23390: A potential agent for mapping cerebral dopamine D-1 receptors. *J. Nucl. Med.* **30,** 931 (abstract).

Muhr C., Bergström M., Lundberg P.O., Bergström K. and Långström B. (1986) In vivo measurement of dopamine receptors in pituitary adenomas using positron emission tomography. *Acta Radiol. Synopsis.* **369**, 406.

Mukherjee J., Luh K.E., Yasillo N., Perry B.D., Levy D., Chin C-T., Ortega C., Beck R.N. and Cooper M. (1990) Dopamine D-2 receptors imaged by PET in Cebus apella using [^{18}F]benzamide neuroleptic. *European J. Parmacol.* **175,** 363.

Pimoule C., Schoemaker H., Reynolds G.P. and Langer S.Z. (1985) ^{3}H-SCH 23390 labelled D1 dopamine receptors are unchanged in schizophrenia and parkinsons disease. *Eur. J. Pharmacol.* **114,** 235.

Raisman R., Cash R., Ruberg M., Javoy-Agid F, Agid Y. (1985) Binding of ^{3}H-SCH 23390 to D1 receptors in the putamen of control and parkinsonian subjects. *Eur. J. Parmacol.* **113**, 467

Ravert. H.T., Wilson. A.A., Dannals R.F., Wong D.F. and Wagner H.N. (1987) Radiosynthesis of a selective dopamine D-1 receptor antagonist: R(+)-7-chloro-8-hydroxy-3-[^{11}C]methyl-1-phenyl-2,3,4,5-tetrahydro-^{1}H-3-benzazepine ([^{11}C]SCH 23390). *Appl. Radiat. Isot.* **38,** 305.

Rinne J.O., Lahinen A., Någren K., Bergman J., Solin O., Haaparanta M., Ruotsalainen U. and Rinne U.K. (1990) PET demonstrates different behaviour of striatal dopamine D-1 and D-2 receptors in early Parkinson's disease. *J. Neurosci. Res.* **27**, 494.

Schultz D.W., Wyrick S.D. and Mailman R.B. (1985) ^{3}H-SCH 23390 has the characteristics of a dopamine receptor ligand in the rat central nervous system. *Eur. J. Parmacol.* **106**, 211

Seeman P., Lee T., Chau-Wong M. and Wong K. (1976) Antipsychotic drug doses and neuroleptic/dopamine receptors. *Nature* **261**,717.

Sedvall G., Farde L., Persson A. and Wiesel F-A. (1986a) Imaging of neurotransmitter receptors in the living human brain. *Arch. Gen. Psychiat.* **43**, 995.

Sedvall G., Farde L., Stone.Elander S. and Halldin C. (1986b) Dopamine D1-receptor binding in the living human brain. In: *Breese G.R., Creese I. (eds) Neurobiology of central D1-dopamine receptors. Plenum, New York,* 119.

Sedvall G., Farde L., Barnett A., Hall H. and Halldin C. (1991) ^{11}C-SCH 39166, a selective ligand for visualization of dopamine D-1 receptor binding in the monkey brain using PET. *Psychopharmacology* **103**, 150.

Suhara T., Fukuda H., Inoue O., Itoh T., Suzuki K., Yamasaki T. and Tateno Y. (1991) Age-related changes in human D1 dopamine receptors measured by positron emission tomography. *Psychopharmacology* **103**, 41.

Waddington J.L. and O'Boyle K.M. (1989) Drugs acting on brain dopamine receptors: a conceptual re-evaluation five years after the first selective D-1 antagonist. *Pharmac. Ther.* **43,** 1.

Wagner H.N., Burns H.D., Dannals R.F., Wong D.F., Långström B., Duelfer T., Frost J.J., Ravert H.T., Links J.M., Rosenblom S.B., Lukas S.E., Kramer A.V. and Kuhar M.J. (1983) Imaging dopamine receptors in the human brain by positron emission tomography. *Science* **221**, 1264.

MONOAMINE PRECURSORS IN PET RESEARCH- BIOCHEMICAL ISSUES AND FUNCTIONAL SIGNIFICANCE

J Tedroff , P Hartvig , H Ågren , P Bjurling , B Långström

Abstract

Aromatic amino acid monoamine precursors can be applied in PET studies to study cerebral uptake of the amino acid neurotransmitter precursors and the subsequent intracerebral synthesis of monoamines. The modification of the intracerebral kinetics induced by the action of aromatic L-amino acid decarboxylase (AADC), a nonspecific enzyme which catalyses the decarboxylation of a large number of aromatic L-amino acids, permits the possibility to interpret kinetic information in terms of a biochemical process *in vivo*. The advantage of studying AADC characteristics *in vivo* is emphasised by the relatively high sensitivity of AADC *in vitro* for changes in the reaction milieu. Several important functional implications can be derived from studying monoamine precursor kinetics *in vivo* with PET.

Introduction

Monoamines such as dopamine and serotonin play important roles in neurotransmission and in the modulation of neurotransmitter release (Carlsson, 1987). Accordingly, disorders in central monoaminergic transmission have been shown, and hypothesized, to be the underlying cause of several clinical disorders. The dopamine deficiency following nigrostriatal degeneration in Parkinson's disease, is well accepted to largely attribute to the muscular rigidity, akinesia and tremor, which are characteristic features of the disease (Agid, 1989). The monoamine hypothesis for the etiology of affective disorders as well as schizophrenia were largely formulated on the basis of pharmacological observations such as on the inhibition of reuptake of serotonin and norepinephrine by tricyclic antidepressive drugs and on the dopamine receptor blocking

J. C. Baron et al. (eds.), Brain Dopaminergic Systems: Imaging with Positron Tomography, 39–52.

action of antipsychotic drugs (Meltzer and Lowy, 1987; Seeman, 1987).

Until now, several aromatic amino acid monoamine precursors have been possible to label with positron emitting radionuclides and applied in PET studies. Among these, the L-DOPA analogue, 6-[^{18}F]fluoro-L-DOPA has been used for a decade (Garnett et al. 1983). More recently several other radiotracers have been developed such as the native precursors of dopamine and serotonin, [^{11}C]-L-DOPA (Tedroff et al. 1991b, Hartvig et al. 1991d) and [^{11}C]-L-5-hydroxy-tryptophan (5HTP) (Hartvig et al. 1991a) respectively. Moreover, the *m*-tyrosine analogue 4-[^{18}F]fluoro-*m*-tyrosine has also been reported to be suitable for PET studies (Melega et al. 1989; Chirakal et al. 1991).

Synthesis of monoamines

Monoamines derived from aromatic L-amino acids are formed by the splitting of carbon dioxide, a reaction first described by Holtz in 1939. In mammals it appears that only two enzymes catalyse the decarboxylation of aromatic amino acids; histidine decarboxylase (EC 4.1.1.22) and aromatic L-amino acid decarboxylase (AADC, EC 4.1.1.28) (for review see Bowsher and Henry, 1986). Unlike histidine decarboxylase, which only catalyses the formation of histamine, AADC is a nonspecific enzyme catalysing the formation of several monoamines including the important neurotransmitters dopamine and serotonin as well as the formation of biogenic amines such as tyramine, phenyletylamine and tryptamine of which functional significance is uncertain. Various α-methyl analogues of these aromatic amino acids are also substrates of AADC to produce "false" transmitters, such as α-methyldopa which is used as an antihypertensive agent (Carlsson, 1987).

AADC is found in the brain were its functional significance is obvious. In the human brain, *in vitro*, the caudate, putamen and the hypothalamus have consistently been shown to exhibit the highest AADC activities (Lloyd and Hornykiewicz, 1972; MacKay et al. 1978; Nagatsu et al. 1979). High AADC activity has also been found in the pineal gland, a tissue rich in melatonin. The cerebral cortex has generally been found to contain very low AADC activity. In tissues such as the cerebellar cortex, cerebral and cerebellar white matter AADC activity has been found very low or abundant. Additionally, in the primate brain the distribution of newly synthesized serotonin and dopamine following administration of the amine precursors 5-hydroxy-tryptophan and L-DOPA *in vivo,* correlates closely to the distribution of AADC found *in vitro* (Lloyd et al. 1975; Tsukada et al. 1975). In the brain, measurable amounts of AADC has also been found on locations where its functional significance is ambiguous, such as in cerebral capillaries, where it is thought to serve as a enzymatic blood-brain barrier (Hardebo et al. 1977).

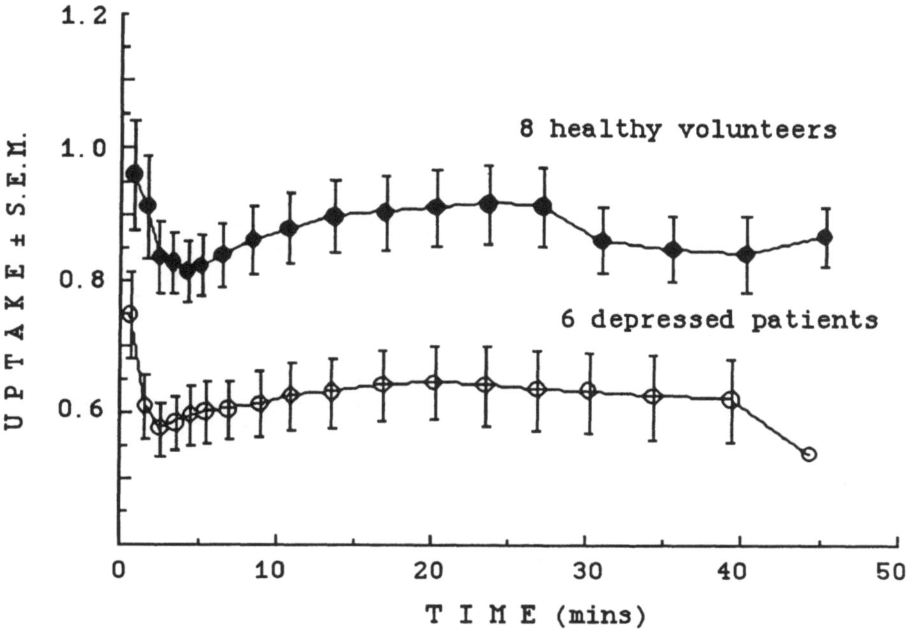

Figure 1. Time-dependent brain uptake of radioactivity normalized to administered radioactivity and body weight after administration of [^{11}C]-L-5-hydroxy-tryptophan in depressed patients and healthy volunteers (from Ågren et al. 1991).

Blood-brain barrier transport

Aromatic L-amino acids are transported into the brain via a carrier-mediated mechanism, the so-called L- (leucine-preferring) system, which is thought to be common for all neutral aromatic and branched-chained amino acids (Oldendorf, 1971). This carrier mechanism is sodium-independent and has been shown to be saturable (Wade and Katzman, 1975, Partridge and Choi, 1986). The carrier has also been suggested to be regulated by a ß-adrenergic mechanism (Eriksson and Carlsson, 1988). Thus, the transport mechanism over the blood-brain barrier (BBB) is regarded as an important site for regulation of amino acid supply into the neurons. Several studies using positron emitter labelled aromatic L-amino acids and PET have been able to demonstrate characteristics of this BBB transport *in vivo* such as saturability and competition with other amino acids for brain uptake (Leenders et al. 1986; Tedroff et al. 1991a, 1991b). Moreover, using [^{11}C]-5HTP and PET, BBB transport of the amino acid has recently been shown to be involved in the depressive pathology (Ågren et al. 1991, figure 1).

Why are aromatic L-amino acid amine precursors retained in the striatum ?

The striatum receives monoamine projection mainly from dopaminergic neurons situated in the midbrain and has therefore high concentrations of dopamine and dopamine synthesizing enzymes (Agid, 1989). In striatal nerve-terminals, endogenously synthesized dopamine is to a great extent concentrated in intracellular granulas by an active process which requires ATP, from where it is available for release by nerve impulses (Carlsson et al. 1962).

The clinical importance of the vesicular monoamine stores is demonstrated by the effects produced by drugs such as the alkaloid reserpine, which has been shown to deplete brain stores of serotonin (Shore et al. 1955), noradrenaline and dopamine (Carlsson et al. 1957). The antipsychotic action of reserpine was reported by Sen and Bose (1931) and the parkinsonism resembling hypokinesia and rigidity induced by reserpine is well established.

However, several lines of evidence suggest that monoamines formed from exogenously administered precursors can be retained in monoaminergic neurons and be functional independently from the vesicular storage pool. In reserpinized animals the build up of striatal dopamine after administration of L-DOPA is similar to that of controls (Melamed, 1988) and in normal rats the increase in striatal dopamine content following administration of L-DOPA is only to a limited extent found in the vesicular pool (Buu, 1989). Moreover, it has long been known that the symptoms of monoamine depletion after reserpine administration can be reversed by exogenously administered L-DOPA and 5HTP (Carlsson et al. 1957). The suggestion of multiple functional monoamine storage pools has further been emphasised by pharmacological evidence (McMillen et al 1980).

The positron emitter labelled aromatic L-amino acid monoamine precursors applied in PET studies, including [^{11}C]-5HTP, have all been shown to preferentially accumulate in the striatum. The importance of the nigrostriatal projection for this retention has been demonstrated after experimental lesions of the nigrostriatal dopamine system such as after administration of the neurotoxin MPTP. Such lesions have been shown to decrease the retention of radioactivity in the striatum after administration of 6-

[^{18}F]fluoro-L-DOPA (Calne et al. 1985), [^{11}C]-L-DOPA (Tedroff et al. 1991b) and [^{11}C]-5HTP (Hartvig et al. 1991a).

Convincing evidence suggest that the decrease in retention following nigrostriatal bundle lesions merely reflects a reduction of AADC activity. The peripheral decarboxylation of an aromatic amino acid has generally been shown to markedly reduce the ability for the resulting amine to penetrate the BBB (Oldendorf, 1971; Melamed et al. 1990; Table 1). Accordingly, the change in the chemical configuration induced by decarboxylation markedly changes the intracerebral kinetics of the resulting amine. Using [^{11}C]-L-DOPA and PET it has recently been shown that administration of [carboxyl-^{11}C]-L-DOPA does not result in specific striatal accumulation of radioactivity since the label is lost as rapidly equilibrating ^{11}C-carbon dioxide after decarboxylation (Tedroff et al. 1991b; Hartvig et al. 1991a). Moreover, in the primate striatum, the rate constant of the kinetic conversion of [ß-^{11}C]-L-DOPA decreases dose-dependently after pretreatment with centrally acting AADC inhibitors (Tedroff et al. 1991b, 1991c). Similar results have also been shown for [^{11}C]-5HTP (Hartvig et al. 1991a). This suggests that the specific striatal accumulation of radioactivity following administration of radiolabelled aromatic L-amino acids grossly indicates decarboxylation of tracer and subsequent retention of the resulting amine. The rate of this kinetic conversion is thus a direct measure of decarboxylation.

TABLE 1. Brain uptake index (BUI) of amino acids and corresponding amines given as percentage of ^{3}HOH reference (from Oldendorf, 1971).

amino acid	BUI	amine	BUI
L-Tyrosine	50	Tyramine	3.07
L-DOPA	20	Dopamine	3.85
DL- 5HTP	7.4	Serotonin	2.6
Histidine	53	Histamine	1.61
Mannitol	1.94		

Methodological considerations

Enzymology

Two parameters are of importance when examining the kinetics of AADC. These are the maximal velocity (V_{max}) which is the amount of product synthesized when the enzymes' active centres are saturated with substrates (amino acid, co-factors), and the Michaelis constant (K_m) which is expressed as the concentration of substrate producing half maximal velocity. The V_{max} and Michaelis constants for L-DOPA and 5HTP have been estimated in numerous studies (Sims et al. 1973; Rahman et al. 1981). Generally, investigations on tissue from several mammalian species have yielded substantially larger values for L-DOPA than for 5HTP. The same appears to be true for human postmortal tissue (Rahman and Nagatsu, 1982). However, the magnitude of the Michaelis constant for most aromatic amino acid substrates have been shown to exceed the endogenous concentration of the aromatic amino acid. This has promoted the speculation that the rate of monoamine synthesis should be first-order thus simplifying the the Michaelis-Menten rate equation to to $V = V_{max}/K_m*[\text{amino acid}]$. This relationship would then be valid when the concentration of the amino acid is well below the Michaelis constant. Using PET and [^{11}C]-L-DOPA it has been shown that injection of pharmacological doses (2-5 mg/kg) in primates and humans yield concentrations in the brain that are several orders in magnitude lower than the Michaelis constants estimated *in vitro*. Moreover, injection of 4 mg/kg L-DOPA/[^{11}C]-L-DOPA in the rhesus monkey did not produce any change in the rate of the kinetic conversion of the tracer in the striatum again supporting the presence of a high Michaelis constant *in vivo*. Thus, saturation of AADC seems unlikely to occur with L-DOPA as substrate, even when administered in pharmacological doses. This is supported by the clinical observation of good correlation between L-DOPA dose and clinical response in Parkinson's disease (Bredberg et al. 1990)

The finding that the Michaelis constant of AADC for 5HTP *in vitro* has generally been estimated lower than that of L-DOPA may indicate that the catalytic site of AADC for 5HTP can be saturated *in vivo* by the administration of high doses 5HTP. To test this hypothesis we have recently assessed striatal [^{11}C]-5HTP retention in non-human primates *in vivo* by PET using tracer doses and pharmacological doses of the amino acid (Hartvig et al. 1991b). It could be shown that pretreatment with 5-6 mg/kg 5HTP markedly decreased the rate constant of the kinetic conversion of [^{11}C]-5HTP in the striatum, which is compatible with self-inhibition of 5HTP at the catalytic site of AADC. This may give a tentative biochemical explanation for the therapeutic failures with high doses of 5HTP in some patients with affective disorders.

Kinetic modelling

The kinetic models used for calculating regional specific utilization of aromatic L-amino acids with PET have generally suggested unidirectional first-order kinetics.

However, this model assumes that the pool of labelled amine and amine metabolites formed after decarboxylation are irreversibly retained in the specific compartment within the measurement time. From a theoretical point of view this is of course misleading. Once the carboxylic group is lost the radiolabel will leave the brain by the following ways: 1. by diffusion of the resulting amine 2. by diffusion or via specific transport systems for the labelled amine metabolites. Until now there has been no attempts to estimate the impact of this efflux on the results obtained from kinetic modelling. However, indirect evidence indicate the unidirectional model being an acceptable approximation. Pharmacological challenges with inhibitors of monoaminoxidase, an enzyme involved in monoamine metabolism, has not been shown to induce measurable alterations in the intracerebral kinetics of several monoamine precursors (Tedroff et al. 1991b; Hartvig et al. 1991a). Moreover, the linearity of the curves obtained from multiple time-uptake graphs generated from PET data using monoamine precursors indicate a reasonable agreement with the postulated model (Martin et al. 1989; Tedroff et al. 1990, 1991b; Brooks et al. 1990; Hartvig et al. 1991a, 1991d).

The appearance of radiolabelled amino acid metabolites in the brain is an additional factor that may produce erratic results when calculating amine precursor uptake data. The rate of appearance of 3-O-methylated metabolites in plasma vary considerably between the different amino acid substrates. After i.v. injection of 6-$[^{18}F]$fluoro-L-DOPA in humans, the ratio of the concentrations in plasma of 3-O-methyl-6-$[^{18}F]$fluoro-L-DOPA to 6-$[^{18}F]$fluoro-L-DOPA increases linearly with time, the O-methylated metabolite exceeding the concentration of 6-$[^{18}F]$fluoro-L-DOPA in plasma 17 minutes after i.v. injection of the radiotracer (Martin et al. 1989). In rats O-methylated 6-$[^{18}F]$fluoro-L-DOPA metabolite levels increase in plasma at a rate greater than $[^{3}H]$-L-DOPA (Melega et al. 1990). Since 3-O-methylDOPA is a poor substrate of AADC (Ferrini and Glaser, 1964) significant contribution of this metabolite to the total radioactive pool in the brain would appearingly decrease the specific utilization by elevating "background" radioactivity. To asses the impact of O-methylated metabolites on the quantitative measures of L-DOPA and fluoro-L-DOPA PET data, we recently compared cerebral kinetics of [ß-^{11}C]-L-DOPA and 6-fluoro-[ß-^{11}C]-L-DOPA in non-human primates after inhibition of catechol-O-methyl transferase (COMT), a nonspecific enzyme which catalyses the O-methylation of catechols (Hartvig et al.1991c). Following COMT inhibition, the apparent rate constant of the striatal kinetic conversion of 6-fluoro-[ß-^{11}C]-L-DOPA increased 60% indicating a substantial decrease in "background" radioactivity. For [ß-^{11}C]-L-DOPA no significant change in this value was measured after COMT inhibition, again supporting the relatively slow slow peripheral O-methylation of this compound. The *m*-tyrosine analogue 4-[^{18}F]fluoro-*m*-tyrosine is a poor substrate of COMT and no 3-O-methylated metabolite was detected in plasma or brain after i.v. injection of this compound (Melega et al. 1989).

Selectivity of AADC

Several approaches have been used to establish whether multiple decarboxylases exist for aromatic amino acids. These include immunotitration experiments (Christenson et al. 1972), immunohistochemical methods (Goldstein et al. 1972) and approaches using administration of neurotoxic agents (Melamed et al. 1980). Although some previous studies indicate the presence of multiple decarboxylases for L-DOPA and 5HTP, convincing evidence is still missing. Still, the AADC protein may contain a complex catalytic site with adjacent binding sites for fixing substrates. For example, saturation of AADC by 5HTP did not significantly decrease the striatal conversion of [ß-^{11}C]-L-DOPA in primates, although the striatal conversion of [^{11}C]-5HTP was markedly reduced (Hartvig et al. 1991b). Therefore, careful phrasing is mandatory when describing monoamine precursor kinetics with PET. For example, the monofluorinated monoamine precursor [^{18}F]fluoro-*m*-tyrosine has recently been suggested to be a "dopaminergic" marker (Chirakal et al. 1991). However, *m*-tyrosine is an excellent substrate of AADC, but does not yield dopamine after decarboxylation. Further, the effect of monofluorination on the substrate-enzyme interaction is not known. Clearly, this issue is not just semantics but touches upon the important question of how to interpret monoamine precursor uptake data. The finding of parallel reductions of [^{11}C]nomifensine binding, a tracer with affinity for the dopamine transporter, and 6-[^{18}F]fluoro-L-DOPA retention in Parkinson's disease (Tedroff et al. 1990) provides indirect evidence for 6-[^{18}F]fluoro-L-DOPA being a marker of the presynaptic integrity of the dopamine system but does not necessarily imply that the tracer demonstrates cerebral L-DOPA kinetics.

Is AADC modulated by neuronal activity ?

It has previously been shown that the activity of tyrosine hydroxylase (TH) is modulated by neuronal activity (Masserano and Weiner, 1983). Under normal conditions TH is nearly saturated and has thus been assumed to be rate-limiting in the sequence of biochemical events that lead to the formation of catecholamines. Based on the finding that AADC under normal condition is subsaturated it has been assumed not to be rate-limiting in the biochemical process of monoamine formation and thus not modulated by neuronal activity (Bowsher and Henry, 1986). Recent evidence indicate that this concept most likely needs a re-evaluation. In the rat retina the V_{max} of AADC for L-DOPA has been shown to increase two-fold after administration of adrenoceptor agonists (Rosetti et al. 1989). Moreover, using PET and [^{11}C]-L-DOPA, the rate constant for the conversion of the radiotracer in the striatum of rhesus monkeys has been shown to increase 60% after pretreatment with 20 mg/kg of 6R-L-erythro-5,6,7,8-tetrahydro-biopterin, a compound which has been shown to increase dopaminergic turnover (Watanabe et al. 1990; Koshimura et al. 1990). The use of radiolabelled AADC inhibitors such as the hydrazine NSD 1015 would be valuable to further clarify the relationship between the amount of AADC molecules and AADC activity *in vivo*.

Comparison of *in vivo* and *in vitro* data.

The measurement of AADC activity *in vitro* has generally been associated with relatively large standard errors in the experimental data (Bowsher and Henry, 1986). To date, PET measurements of the activity of AADC *in vivo* for various substrates such as [^{11}C]-L-DOPA, [^{11}C]-5HTP and [^{18}F]fluoro-L-DOPA has been carried out by several groups.

From Table 2 it is evident that AADC measurements *in vitro* from postmortal tissue are generally associated with higher standard errors in the experimental data. This variation has been postulated to be due to postmortal instability of the enzyme although this has not been proved (MacKay, 1978). Additionally, it is well known that individual *in vitro* decarboxylation rates are highly influenced by reaction parameters such as pH, the presence of exogenous pyridoxal-5-phosphate (PLP) and organic solvents (Bowsher and Henry, 1986). Based on the foregoing, it seems resonable to assume that more reliable results are obtained when studying AADC properties *in vivo*. This may explain the smaller variations in the experimental data obtained with PET. The recent indications of a coupling between AADC activity and monoaminergic turnover further emphasises the importance of standardized protocols when examining AADC kinetics.

TABLE 2. Comparison of results obtained from AADC activity estimations for the caudate nucleus using L-DOPA and 5HTP as substrates *in vivo* and *in vitro*.

In vivo

Method	Species/ number	Substrate ± S.E.M	Rate constant[a]	CV[b]
PET[1]	H/10	[^{11}C]-L-DOPA	0.0151±0.0025	16%
PET[2]	H/30	[^{18}F]-L-FDOPA	0.0107±0.0019	18%
PET[3]	Rhe/10	[^{11}C]-L-DOPA	0.0105±0.0004	4%
PET[4]	Rhe/5	[^{11}C]-5HTP	0.0056±0.0008	14%

In vitro

Method	Species/ number	Substrate ±S.E.M	AADC activity[c]	CV
HPLC[5]	H/6	L-DOPA	8.60±5.06	59%
Radiometric[6]	H/14	DL-DOPA[carboxyl^{14}C]	366±103	28
HPLC[7]	H/4	L-DOPA	227±65.3	29%
HPLC[7]	H/4	5HTP	28.7±8.7	30%

Data is taken from the following references: [1]Hartvig et al. 1991d [2]Brooks et al. 1990 [3]Tedroff et al. 1991 [4]Hartvig et al. 1991a [5]Nagatsu et al. 1979 [6]Lloyd and Hornykiewicz, 1972 [7]Rahman and Nagatsu, 1982

[a]denotes the unidirectional rate constant (min^{-1}) of the kinetic conversion of the amine precursor induced by decarboxylation. [b]CV-coefficient of variation, calculated as S.E.M/mean. [c]Amount decarboxylated per time and tissue unit, absolute values vary with the incubation methods used. H-human, Rhe-rhesus monkey

References

Agid Y. (1989) Dopaminergic systems in Parkinson's disease. In: Quinn NP, Jenner PG, eds. Disorders of Movement: Clinical, Pharmacological and Physiological aspects. Academic Press, London, pp. 85-107

Bowsher RR, Henry DP. (1986) Aromatic L-amino acid decarboxylase: biochemistry and functional significance. In: Boulton AA, Baker GB, Yu PH, eds. Neuromethods, Series 1: Neurochemistry. Humana Press, Clifton, New Jersey, pp. 33-77

Bredberg E, Tedroff J, Aquilonius S-M, Paalzow L. (1990) Pharmacokinetics and effects of levodopa in advanced Parkinson's disease. Eur J Clin Pharmacol 39:385-389
Buu N. (1989) Vesicular accumulation of dopamine following L-DOPA administration. Biochem Pharmacol 38:1787-1792
Calne DB, Langston JW, Martin WRW et al. (1985) Positron emission tomography after MPTP: observations relating to the cause of Parkinson's disease. Nature 317:246-248
Carlsson A, Hillarp N-Å, Waldeck B. (1962) A Mg^{2+}-ATP dependent storage mechanism in the amine granules of the adrenal medulla. Med Exp. 6:47-53
Carlsson A, Lindqvist M, Magnusson T. (1957) 3,4-Dihydroxyphenylalanine and 5-hydroxytryptophan as reserpine antagonists. Nature 180:1200
Carlsson A, Rosengren E, Bertler Å, Nilsson J. (1957) Effect of reserpine on the metabolism of catechol amines. In: Garattini S, Ghetti V eds. Psychotropic drugs, Elsevier, Amsterdam, pp. 363-372
Carlsson A. (1987) Monoamines in the central nervous system: A historical perspective. In: Meltzer HY ed. Psychopharmacology: The third generation of progress. Raven Press, New York, pp. 39-48
Chirakal R, Garnett ES, Schrobilgen GJ, Nahmias C, Firnau G. (1991) ^{18}F and the dopamine pathway. Chem Brit 14:47-52
Christenson JG, Dairman W, Undenfriend S. (1972) On the identity of DOPA decarboxylase and 5-HTP decarboxylase. Proc Natl Acad Sci USA 69:343-374
Eriksson T, Carlsson A. (1988) ß-adrenergic control of brain uptake of large neutral amino acids. Life Sci 42:1583-1589
Garnett ES, Firnau G, Nahmias C, Chirakal R. (1983) Striatal dopamine metabolism in living monkeys examined by positron emission tomography. Brain Res 280:169-171
Goldstein M, Fuxe K, Hökfelt T. (1972) Characterisation and tissue localization of catecholamine-syntheseizing enzymes. Pharmacol Rev 24:293-295
Hardebo JE, Edvinsson L, Owman C, Rosengren E. (1977) Quantitative evaluation of the blood-brain barrier capacity to form dopamine from circulating L-DOPA. Acta Physiol Scand 99:377-384
Hartvig P , Tedroff J, Lundqvist H, Bjurling P, Långström B. (1991a) Brain kinetics of ^{11}C-labelled tryptophan and 5-hydroxy-tryptophan in the brain of the Rhesus monkey measured with positron emission tomography. Submitted to J Neural Transm
Hartvig P, Lindner KJ, Tedroff J, Bjurling P, Chang Chi-Wei, Tsukada H, Watanabe Y, Långström B. (1991b) Positron emission tomographic studies on the selectivity and saturation of 5-hydroxy-L-tryptophan decarboxylase in the monkey brain. Submitted to J Neural Transm

Hartvig P, Lindner KJ, Tedroff J, Bjurling P, Hörnfelt K, Långström B. (1991c) Regional brain kinetics of 6-fluoro-[^{11}C]-L-DOPA and [^{11}C]-L-DOPA following COMT inhibition. A study in vivo using PET. Submitted to J Neural Transm

Hartvig P, Ågren H, Reibring L, Tedroff J, Bjurling P, Kihlberg T, Långström B. (1991d) Brain kinetics of [ß-^{11}C]-L-DOPA in humans studied by positron emission tomography. J Neural Transm (in press)

Holz P. (1939) Dopadecarboxylase. Naturwissenschaften 27:724-725

Koshimura K, Miwa S, Lee K, Fujiwara M, Watanabe Y. (1990) Enhancement of dopamine release in vivo from the rat striatum by dialytic perfusion of 6R-L-erythro-5,6,7,8-tetrahydro-biopterin. J Neurochem 54:1391-1397

Leenders KL, Poewe WH, Palmer AJ, Brenton DP, Frackowiak RSJ. (1986) Inhibition of L-[^{18}F]fluorodopa uptake into human brain by amino acids demonstrated by positron emission tomography. Ann Neurol 20:258-262

Lloyd KG, Davidson L, Hornykiewicz O. (1975) The neurochemistry of Parkinson's disease: effect of L-DOPA therapy. J Pharmacol Exp Ther 195:453-464

Lloyd KG, Hornykiewicz O. (1972) Occurrence and distribution of aromatic L-amino acid (L-dopa) decarboxylase in the human brain. J Neurochem 19:1549-1559

MacKay AVP, Davies P, Dewar AJ, Yates CM. (1978) Regional distribution of enzymes associated with neurotransmission by monoamines, acetylcholine and GABA in the human brain. J Neurochem 30:827-839

Martin WRW, Palmer MR, Patlak CS, Calne DM. (1989) Nigrostriatal function in humans studied with positron emission tomography. Ann Neurol 26:453-464

Masserano JM, Weiner N. (1983) Tyrosine hydroxylase regulation in the central nervous system. Mol Cell Biochem 53:129-152

Mc Millen BA, German DC, Shore PA. (1980) Functional and pharmacological significance of brain dopamine and norepinephrine storage pools. Biochem Pharm 29:3045-3050

Melamed E, Hefti F, Wurtman RJ. (1980) DOPA and 5-HTP decarboxylase activities in rat striatum: effect of selective destruction of dopaminergic or serotoninergic input. J Neurochem 34:1753-1756

Melamed E, Rosenthal J, Reches A. (1990) Systemically administered dopamine: can it cross the blood-brain barrier after inhibition of monoamine oxidase ? Abstract. European Conference on Parkinson's disease and Extrapyramidal disorders

Melamed E. (1988) Role of the nigrostriatal dopaminergic neurons in mediating the effect of exogenous L-dopa in Parkinson's disease. Mount Sinai J Med 55:35-42

Melega WP, Luxen A, Perlmutter MM, Nissenson C, Phelps M, BarrioJR. (1990) Comparative in vivo metabolism of 6-[^{18}F]fluoro-L-DOPA and [^{3}H]L-DOPA in rats. Biochem Pharmacol 39:1853-1860

Melega WP, Perlmutter MM, Luxen A, Nissenson HK, Grafton ST, Huang S-C, Phelps ME, Barrio JR. 4-[^{18}F]Fluoro-L-*m*-tyrosine: an L-3,4-dihydroxyphenylalanine analog for probing presynaptic dopaminergic function with positron emission tomography. J Neurochem 1989;53:311-314

Melzer HY, Lowy MT. (1987) The serotonin hypothesis of depression. In: Meltzer HY, ed. Psychopharmacology: Third generation of progress. Raven Press, New York, pp. 513-516

Nagatsu T, Kato T, Nagatsu I et al. (1979) Catecholamine-related enzymes in the brain of patients with parkinsonism and Wilson's disease. In: Poirier LJ, Sourkes TL, Bédard PJ eds. Advances in Neurology, Raven Press, New York, pp. 283-292

Oldendorf WH. (1971) Brain uptake of radiolabeled amino acids, amines, and hexoses after arterial injection. Am J Physiol 221:1629-1639

Partridge WM, Choi TB. (1986) Neutral amino acid transport at the blood-brain-barrier. Fed Proc 45:2073-2078

Rahman MK, Nagatsu T, Kato T. (1981) Aromatic L-amino acid decarboxylase activity in central and peripheral tissues and serum of rats with DOPA and 5HTP as substrates. Biochem Pharmacol 30:645-649

Rahman MK, Nagatsu T. (1982) Demonstration of aromatic L-amino acid decarboxylase activity in human brain with L-DOPA and L-5-hydroxytryptophan as substrates by high-performance liquid chrmatography with electrochemical detection. Neurochem Int 4:1-6

Rosetti ZL, Silvia CP, Krajnc D, Neff NH, Hadjiconstantinou M. (1989) Modulation of aromatic L-amino acid decarboxylase via a_2-adrenoceptors. J Neurochem 52:647-652

Seeman P. (1987) Dopamine receptors and the dopamine hypothesis of schizophrenia. Synapse 1:133-152

Sen G, Bose KC. (1931) Rauwolfia serpentina, a new Indian drug for insanity and high blood pressure. Indian Med World 2:194-201

Shore PA, Silver SL, Brodie BD. (1955) Interaction of reserpine on serotonin and lysergic acid diethylamide in brain. Science 122:284-285

Sims KL, Davies GA, Bloom FE. (1973) Activities of DOPA and 5HTP decarboxylases in rat brain: Assay characteristics and distribution. J Neurochem 20:449-464

Tedroff J, Aquilonius S-M, Hartvig P, Bredberg E, Bjurling P, Långström B. (1991a) Cerebral uptake and utilization of [ß-^{11}C]-L-DOPA in Parkinson's disease measured by

positron emission tomography – relations to motor response. Acta Neurol Scand (in press)
Tedroff J, Aquilonius S-M, Hartvig P, Lundqvist H, Bjurling P, Långström B. (1991b) Estimation of regional cerebral utilization of [^{11}C]-L-3,4-dihydroxyphenylalanine (DOPA) in the primate by positron emission tomography. Acta Neurol Scand (in press)
Tedroff J, Aquilonius S-M, Laihinen A, Rinne U, Hartvig P, Andersson J, Lundqvist H, Haaparanta M, Solin O, Antoni G, Gee A D, Ulin J, Långström B. (1990) Striatal kinetics of [^{11}C]-(+)-nomifensine and 6-[^{18}F]fluoro-L-dopa in Parkinson's disease measured with positron emission tomography. Acta Neurol Scand 81:24-30.
Tedroff J, Hartvig P, Bjurling P, Andersson Y, Antoni G, Långström B. (1991c) Central action of benserazide after COMT inhibition demonstrated in vivo by PET. J Neural Transm (in press)
Tsukada Y, Kishimoto H, Nagai K. (1975) Studies on amine metabolism in the monkey brain after administration of amine precursor. Contemporary Primatology, Karger, Basel, pp. 56-66
Wade LA, Katzman R. (1975) Synthetic amino acids and the nature of L-DOPA transport at the blood-brain barrier. J Neurochem 25:837-842
Watanabe Y, Hartvig P, Tedroff J et al. (1991) Elevation of ^{11}C-dopamine turnover in vivo by peripheral administration of 6R-tetrahydrobiopterin in monkey striatum. In: Bleu et al. eds. Pteridine and related biogenic amines in neuropsychiatry, pediatrics and immunology. (in press)
Ågren H, Reibring L, Hartvig P, Tedroff J, Bjurling P, Hörnfelt K, Andersson Y, Lundqvist H, Långström B. (1991) Low brain uptake of L-(^{11}C)-5-hydroxytryptophan in major depression. A positron emission tomography study on patients and healthy volunteers. Acta Psychiat Scand (in press)

QUANTITATION PROBLEMS IN POSITRON EMISSION TOMOGRAPHY (PET) AS APPLIED TO THE KINETIC ANALYSIS OF THE STRIATUM DOPAMINE DATA

L. ERIKSSON

H. HERZOG

A.-L. NORDSTRÖM

ABSTRACT. Quantitative determination of striatal dopamine receptor characteristics can be performed with PET. To make a correct interpretation of data, it is of importance to realize the limitations of the technique. In the present paper we discuss the implications of instrumental limitations on the accuracy of the determination of the four rate constants of a three-compartment model. Two different tracers have been tried [^{18}F]-FDG and [^{11}C]-raclopride. With a resolution independent choice of region-of-interest, mainly K1 is affected when structures like the putamen and the caudate are investigated with different spatial resolution, implying that receptor characteristics may be determined with sufficient accuracy with different PET systems and different generations of PET-systems. Errors in cross-calibration between the PET scanner and the well-counter/radiation detector for the determination of the input function also mainly affect K1. Dispersion in automatic blood-sampling systems has minor influence on all rate constants.

1. Introduction

Positron emission tomography (PET) has proven to be a valuable tool in providing functional information of the brain and of other organs. By bolus administrations of labeled tracers, the regional tracer uptake can be analyzed in terms of tracer kinetic models by which functional processes can be described. We can thus determine metabolism and receptor characteristics of the brain and the heart. The radionuclides commonly used are the "bio-isotopes" ^{18}F, ^{13}N, ^{11}C and ^{15}O. This paper concerns PET studies of small structures of the human brain, such as the striatum. The tracer kinetic model (compartment model) applied to the kinetic analysis of radioligand binding has been developed as an extension of the Sokoloff model for deoxyglucose (Sokoloff et al 1977, Phelps et al 1979, Mintun et al 1984, Wong et al 1986, Huang et al 1987). The model predicts the following differential equations:

J. C. Baron et al. (eds.), Brain Dopaminergic Systems: Imaging with Positron Tomography, 53–64.

$$\frac{dC_f}{dt} = K_1C_p - k_2C_f - k_3C_f + k_4C_b \tag{1}$$

$$\frac{dC_b}{dt} = k_3C_f - k_4C_b \tag{2}$$

K_1,k_2,k_3 and k_4 are first order rate constants, K_1 with the dimension (ml/g/min) and k_2,k_3 and k_4 (1/min). The rate constant, k_3, is the product of the bimolecular association rate constant, kon (ml/pmol/min), and the concentration of available receptors (B_{max} - C_b/SA). Bmax is the density of receptors (pmol/ml) and SA is the specific activity of the labeled ligand (Ci/mmol). k_4 is the unimolecular dissociation rate constant, k_{off}. Assuming SA to be high, k_3 is constant with time and we can solve C_f and C_b in terms of the four rate constants and the plasma input function C_p, giving the tissue model prediction:

$$C_{model} = C_f + C_b = f(C_p,K_1,k_2,k_3,k_4) \tag{3}$$

The observed tissue activity , C_{pet}, of the brain is then compared to the model prediction in a least squares sense:

$$(C_{pet}-C_{model})^2 = \text{minimum} \tag{4}$$

We have limited the discussion to the case when k_3 is constant with time and investigated the influence of instrumental limitations on the tracer kinetic constants K_1,k_2,k_3 and k_4.

1.1 OUTLINE OF THE PAPER

For PET determination of bio-chemical parameters, two observations are used, the regional time-activity uptake curve and the time-activity plasma curve, the input function. The kinetic constants are then solved by comparing model data with experimental data in a least squares sense (see equation (4)). Regarding the PET scanner itself, the effect on the determined rate constants due to resolution limitations and errors due to incorrect corrections of absorption, scatter and random coincidences must be considered. In this paper we only discuss the effects due to unresolved structures and the influence of scatter. Partial volume effects or resolution effects will imply that in selected regions-of-interest (ROI:s) of structures smaller than the resolution of the scanner, data will be underestimated(Hoffman et al., 1979). On the other hand, surrounding tissue data will "spill-over" inadequate information into the selected ROI, possibly giving an admixture concealing the true data. We have investigated the effect of different image resolutions on the uptake data and on the analysis of time-activity data in terms of the standard three compartment models with four rate constants. The PET scanners used are a Scanditronix PC4096-15WB whole body system (Rota Kops et al., 1990) and two Scanditronix brain systems, PC2048-15B and PC384-7B (Litton et al. 1990, Litton et al.1984) .

To simulate the situation with different PET scanner resolutions, the cut-off frequency of the reconstruction filter was varied or different Gaussian image filters were applied to a high resolution image. Two different tracers were studied, [^{18}F]-FDG, and [^{11}C]-raclopride to give examples of two tracers with different kinetic properties.

The input function, usually the tracer concentration in arterial plasma as a function of time, must be accurately determined. Automated and/or manual blood sampling techniques can be used (Eriksson et al. 1988). The transfer function that converts the input function to the experimental PET observation gives the physiological information. If compartment models are considered , the model prediction is given by the input function convoluted with a sum of exponential functions. It is obvious that a correct model prediction can only be computed from a correct input function. In this paper we discuss the effect of calibration errors between the blood sampling system and the PET camera, dispersion of the input function and the effect of errors in the time shift between the PET time-activity curve and the input function.

2. Effects due to limitations of the PET-systems

2.1. [^{18}F]-FDG STUDIES

The FDG data was accumulated for 60 minutes. The selected ROI:s were determined from images based on data summation from 30 to 60 minutes. The ROI:s were defined by the total cortex and the right caudate nucleus. The uptake data were decreased of up to 20% when the resolution was changed from 5.5 mm to 11 mm FWHM for the caudate nucleus (Table 1). Thus, functional data such as metabolic data or receptor characteristics may differ between different PET groups if their PET cameras differ in spatial resolution.

For the dynamic analysis of data, time activity curves up to 60 minutes were used. Both the image resolution (FWHM) and the ROI definition were used as variables. For the analysis of the cortical FDG data an individual cortical ROI at an iso-contour level of 60% was defined. A ROI defined in this way will obviously become larger for lower resolution images due to the lower noise. The fitting procedure also included a determination of the blood volume fraction and the time shift between the input function and the tissue data. The results are summarized in Table 2. A 30% increase of the rate constant k2 was found when the image resolution changed from 5.5 to 11 mm, whereas K_1 was nearly constant. CBV decreased with lower resolution and larger ROI:s, possibly due to an increase in the fraction of white matter tissue included with lower resolution. The results were only slightly different when a small fixed ROI was used, defined in the image with the best resolution of 5.5 mm at the iso-contour level of 60% (Table 2b).

Over the right caudate nucleus a ROI was delineated in three different ways: first, a fixed circular ROI with a radius of 8 mm covering the whole structure was chosen; second, a ROI at an iso-contour level of 60% and, third, a ROI at an iso-contour level of 70%. Here again the iso-contour ROI:s had different sizes according to different noise properties at different image resolutions. Because of the small ROI size over the caudate nucleus and the low count rate recorded, the time-activity curves contained considerable noise. Therefore, it was decided to reduce the number of variables to be fitted and to use fixed values of CBV(5%) and time shift (18 sec). As shown in table 3, the rate constants K1 to k3 were found to be different depending on the definition of the ROIs and the image resolution. Only k4 was not affected with results approaching zero. The rate constant k2 decreased for the 60% ROIs, but increased for the 70% ROIs and for the circular ROIs when the image resolution became degraded. Whereas the uptake values may change either in positive or negative direction, the rate constants, except for K1 that always follows the trend of the uptake values, may not reflect this change.

The results obtained in these examples demonstrate that both uptake as and kinetic data are strongly influenced by image resolution and by ROI definition. All rate constants and not only K1, which is directly proportional to the FDG tissue activity, may be affected. Here effects of tissue heterogeneity can be involved, since the variation of image resolution and ROI size yields a different mixture of neighboring tissue, each of which has its own set of rate constants. Another reason may be differences in noise present in the time-activity curves together with difficulties with local minima in the least squares minimization.

2.2. [^{11}C]-RACLOPRIDE

2.2.1 *Spatial resolution effects*. Complementary studies were performed with [^{11}C]-raclopride of high specific activity to give a k_3 constant in time. Only the putamen data were considered. All ROI:s were delineated based on the PET images. To compare the effects of different spatial resolution, fixed ROI:s were used, defined in the image with the highest resolution. The results from this study is shown in Figure 1. When the resolution was changed from 4.5 mm to around 13 mm FHWM, only K1 changed significantly. This was expected since K1 directly reflects the uptake values. The changes in the other rate constants are not significant.

2.2.2 *Spill-over effects*. To investigate the effect of "spill-over", we first modified the analyzing program so that a fraction "f" of admixed white matter data could be included:

$$C_{pet}(\text{putamen}) = C_{model}*(1-f) + f* C_{pet}(\text{white matter}) \qquad (5)$$

where C_{model} is the three compartment model, four parameter prediction and C_{pet} are the measured PET uptake data for the putamen and white matter. A fixed blood volume fraction of 4% was used. The fraction "f" was added as a fifth parameter in the analysis. Studies of the uptake of [^{11}C]-raclopride in the same volunteer investigated with two different brain cameras, PC384-7B and PC2048-15B, were used. The analyses of data are shown in table 4. Except for K_1, the rate constants are in very good agreement showing the excellent compatibility of the two systems. The difference in K_1 is somewhat surprising since a higher K_1 was expected with the higher resolution . However, this difference may reflect either differences in the cross-calibration between the blood sampling systems and the PET scanners or a 20% blood flow decrease between the two different measurements. The fraction "f" found by the program for estimated white matter tissue in the selected putamen ROI is 1.3±0.8 % for the PC2048-15B data and 0.5±0.1% for the PC384-7B. It is surprising that the obtained fractions are so small since we would expect a 10% spill-over of white matter into the putamen, at least in the putamen data from the PC384-7B system. The rate constants, however, are relatively insensitive to admixtures of white matter into the putamen data. This can be seen from Figure 2, where we added different fractions of white matter time-activity data into the putamen time-activity data and analyzed the composite data with the standard three compartment four parameter model with a fixed blood volume of 0.04. Only the decrease in K_1 is significant up to an admixed fraction of white matter data of 20%.

2.2.3. *Effect of scatter*. A profile across the putamen area with and without scatter correction is shown in Figure 3 for a $[^{11}C]$-raclopride study using the Scanditronix PC2048-15B. Without scatter corrections, the time-activity data points for the selected ROI increase with approximately 7%. The rate constants determined with and without scatter corrections are in good agreement except for K_1, which is 8.5% higher with no scatter corrections. This is expected, since the scatter distribution adds a certain fraction of counts to each data point in the time activity curve. This increase of the PET time-activity curve is reflected directly in a proportional increase of K_1.

3. Limitations due to blood sampling

As mentioned in the introduction, the determination of the input function is as important for accurate quantitation as the camera measurement itself. Blood sampling is commonly performed by either manual blood sampling or automated blood sampling techniques (Eriksson et al. 1988). Manual samples are difficult to take when very sharp bolus injections are employed, necessitating a sample rate of 3-5 seconds per sample in the beginning. Automated sampling systems (ABSS) are simpler to use and have the additional advantage of reducing radiation exposure for the personnel. However, catheters used in the automated blood sampling systems give dispersion effects.

For studies with $[^{11}C]$-raclopride, we mix the two techniques by using automated sampling the first five minutes and then manual sampling for the rest of the study. For manual samples a well-counter is used. During the automatic blood sampling period a few additional manual samples may be taken to cross-calibrate the radiation detector of the ABSS, the well-counter and the positron camera.

3.1 EFFECT OF CALIBRATION ERRORS

Investigation of errors in calibration between the blood curve and the PET uptake curves have shown that only the rate constant K_1 is affected. If the input function is underestimated, the model compensates the high tissue activity in the positron camera data by increasing K_1. If dispersion is neglected we overestimate K_1. The detectors with which the input function is determined, must be correctly calibrated against the positron camera. The time phase of the input function relative the PET uptake data must also be accurately known, for a correct comparison between experimental data and model predictions. An illustration of the effect of the time shifts between uptake PET data and the plasma curve is given in figure 4. The figure is based on data from the first three minutes of the raclopride study with cbv kept constant (0.04) and shows that a choice of 15 sec is optimal. However, for a full length study of more than 50 minutes a small time shift of the order of 5 - 10 seconds will not change the calculated rate constants. Actually, no change was found in the rate constants K_1, k_2, k_3, k_4 in this particular study for time shifts of 4 - 21 seconds.

3.2 EFFECT OF DISPERSION

Concerning dispersion in the ABSS system, we have investigated the tissue response in a CBV study with $[^{11}C]$-CO with time frames of 5 seconds during the first two minutes. The ABSS system was used to sample arterial blood from the brachial artery during the same study in order to compare the "grey matter" response with the ABSS blood curve. These are shown in Figure 5a. It is obvious that the ABSS curve is substantially degraded due to dispersion. We have tried a deconvolution assuming an exponential dispersion function with a time constant of 6 seconds. In Figure 5b the deconvoluted ABSS curve is compared with the "grey matter" response. This is composed of an arterial fraction, a capillary fraction and a venous fraction, but should not be too far from the desired arterial input sensed by tissue (Greitz 1956 and personal communication). For $[^{11}C]$-raclopride, deconvolution of the plasma curve results in a slight decrease in all rate constants: K1 with 3%, k2 and k3 with 6%, and k4 with less than 2%.

4. Conclusions

In this paper we have studied the effect of different instrumental errors on the rate constants determined in $[^{18}F]$-FDG and in a few $[^{11}C]$-raclopride studies, the latter with high specific activity. It was found that essentially only K_1 is affected by instrumental errors such as unresolved structures and errors in the cross-calibration between the PET camera itself, the well-counter for manual blood- and plasma samples and the radiation detector of the ABSS. Comparing the uptake of $[^{11}C]$-raclopride in the same volunteer measured in two different PET systems showed that the data are in excellent agreement with the exception of the K_1. Therefore data presented in terms of rate constants can be compared between different PET systems. With systems with different resolutions, however, the ROI:s are defined in different ways. As demonstratedwith FDG, this may also lead to differences in the k_2,k_3 and k_4. For ROI: definitions based on anatomical data from for ex CT or MRI, however, only K_1 may be affected. Since the 3-compartments fits can instable it is usually better to define a larger region to give the time-activity curve, a ROI perhaps covering the full anatomical extent of the structure studied. The resulting time-activity curve will then have data points with better statitistical properties than for a smaller ROI giving perhaps higher accuracy but with much lower precision. A larger ROI delineation may also be motivated by our finding that $[^{11}C]$-raclopride putamen data are relatively insensitive to white matter spill-over. The resulting time activity curves can then be corrected by multiplying the data points with a suitable recovery factor.

5. Tables.

TABLE 1. $[^{18}F]$-FDG activity data in nCi/cc as a function of image resolution

Image resolution	5.5 mm	7 mm	11mm
Cortex	734	658	623
Caudate nucleus	875	768	711

TABLE 2. Results from 3-compartment fits of cortical [^{18}F]-FDG time-activity curves as a function of image resolution.

a) 60% iso-contour ROI individually defined for each FWHM

FWHM(mm)	K1	k2	k3	k4	CBV (%)	Shift (sec)
5.5	0.132	0.303	0.148	0.0132	8.5	17.7
7	0.134	0.344	0.156	0.0139	7.7	17.7
9	0.133	0.361	0.156	0.0131	7.3	17.7
11	0.133	0.393	0.162	0.0140	6.8	17.5

b) 60% iso-contour ROI defined for FWHM = 5.5 mm

FWHM(mm)	K1	k2	k3	k4	CBV (%)	Shift (sec)
5.5	0.132	0.303	0.148	0.0132	8.5	17.7
7	0.131	0.332	0.154	0.0137	8.0	17.8
9	0.132	0.347	0.157	0.0140	7.6	18.1
11	0.132	0.384	0.166	0.0150	7.1	18.1

TABLE 3. Results from a 3-compartment fit of [^{18}F]-FDG caudate time-activity curves as a function of image resolution.

a) Circular ROI with an area of 240 mm^2

FWHM(mm)	K1	k2	k3	k4	CBV (%) fixed	Shift (sec) fixed	mean activity in ROI (nCi/ml)
5.5	0.079	0.154	0.086	0.004	5	18	322
7	0.078	0.170	0.091	0.004	5	18	307
9	0.078	0.177	0.090	0.003	5	18	302
11	0.074	0.175	0.090	0.003	5	18	283

b) 60% iso-contour ROI individually defined for each FWHM

FWHM(mm)	K1	k2	k3	k4	CBV (%) fixed	Shift (sec) fixed	mean activity in ROI (nCi/ml)
5.5	0.103	0.185	0.098	0.00	5	18	425
7	0.094	0.191	0.097	0.00	5	18	376
9	0.084	0.169	0.098	0.00	5	18	367
11	0.074	0.132	0.070	0.00	5	18	326

c) 70% iso-contour ROI individually defined for each FWHM

FWHM(mm)	K1	k2	k3	k4	CBV (%) fixed	Shift (sec) fixed	mean activity in ROI (nCi/ml)
5.5	0.083	0.069	0.049	0.00	5	18	478
7	0.092	0.128	0.074	0.00	5	18	415
9	0.077	0.121	0.087	0.00	5	18	395
11	0.077	0.139	0.076	0.00	5	18	354

TABLE 4. Analysis of spill-over fractions in the putamen data obtained with the PC384-7B and PC2048-15B for the same volunteer.

camera type	K1	k2	k3	k4	fraction white matter
PC2048-15B	0.134	0.303	0.341	0.129	fixed =0
	0.134	0.303	0.340	0.129	0.013±0.008
PC384-7B	0.180	0.322	0.341	0.121	fixed =0
	0.178	0.299	0.326	0.124	0.005±0.001

6. Figures

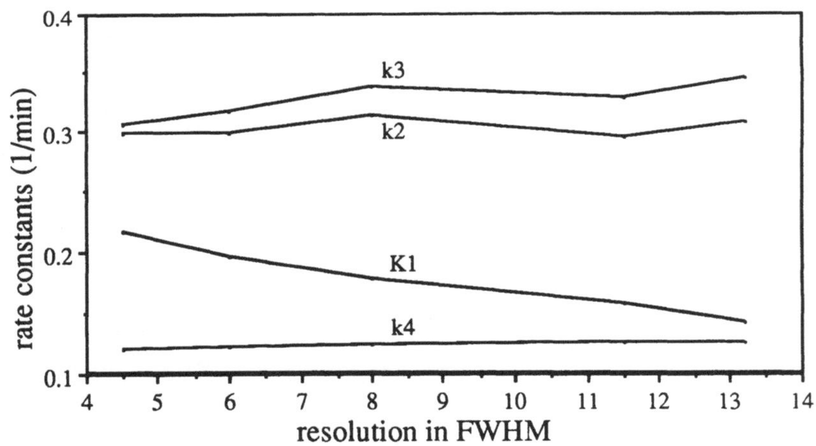

Fig 1. Variations of the [^{11}C]-raclopride rate constants as a function of the image resolution.

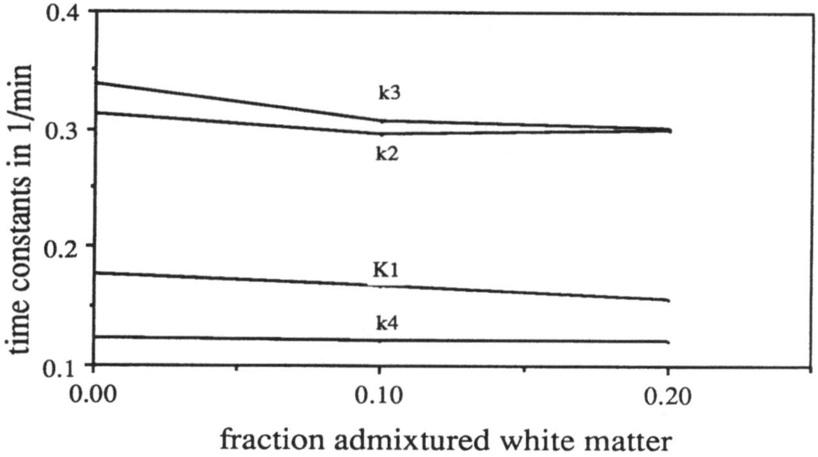

Fig 2. The effect of admixture of white matter time-activity data into putamen data. Only K1 is significantly changed when the fraction white matter is increased.

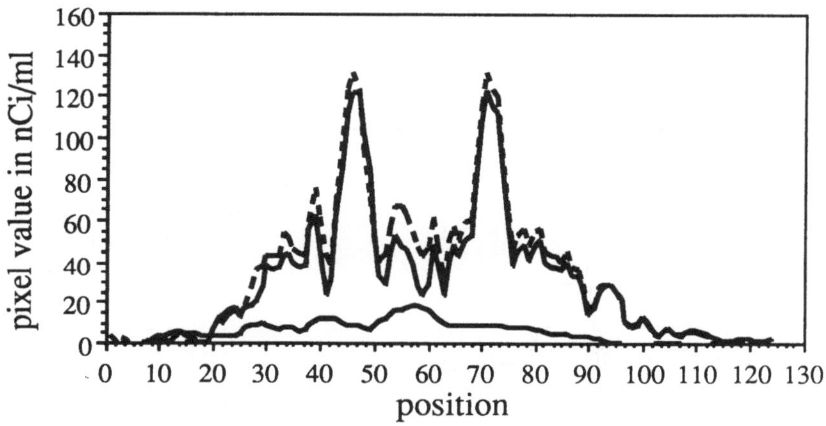

Fig. 3 A profile over a [^{11}C]-raclopride image over the putamen region, with and without scatter corrections obtained with the Scanditronix PC2048-15B camera.

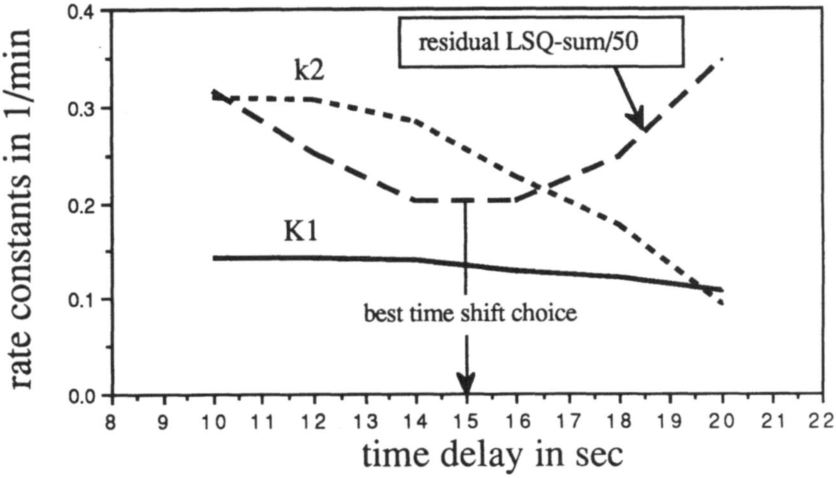

Fig 4. Time shift search between the input function and PET uptake data. For this search only the first 3 minutes have been used to increase the sensitivity. For the full length of the study of 50 minutes, the rate constants do not change appreciably between 4 - 21 seconds. A crude search with a ± 5 second accuracy is thus sufficient.

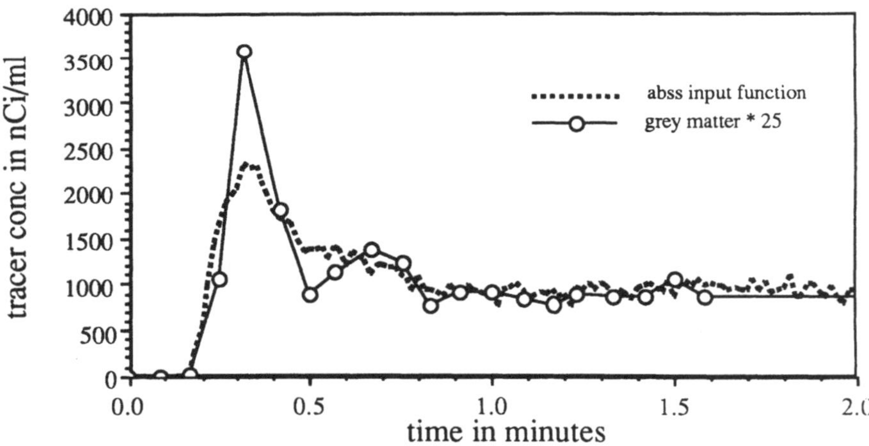

Fig 5a. The figure shows the time-activity curve from a large "grey matter" ROI following injection of [^{11}C]-CO in an attempt to determine the input function actually sensedby the brain tissue. As a comparison, the blood curve measured in the brachial artery parallel to the automated blood sampling system is shown. From the differences, an estimate of the dispersion of the ABSS blood curve can be made.

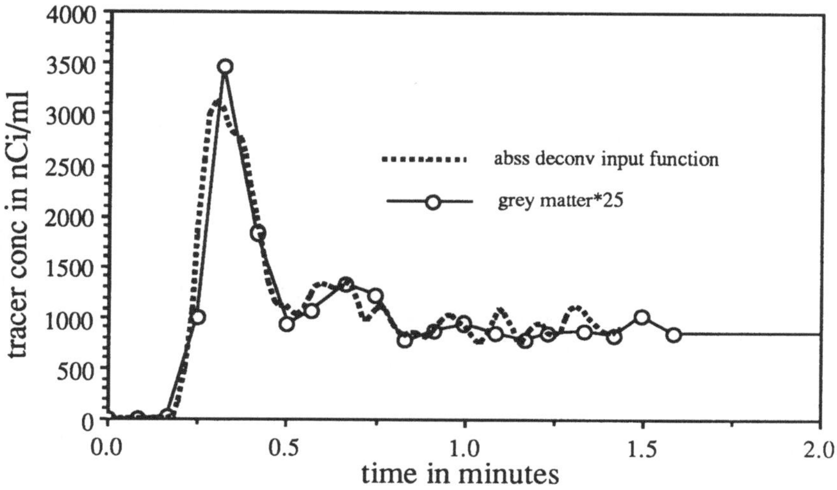

Fig 5b. The same figure as before but with the ABSS blood curve deconvoluted with an exponential dispersion function with a time constant of 6 sec or $10 min^{-1}$.
The agreement between the "grey matter" response and the abss blood curve is now better indicating a dispersion of this order. The effect of a deconvoluted blood curve with this time constant gave a reduction of all rate constants from 2 % to 6%, i.e. well within un expected uncertainty of 10-20 % .

Acknowledgement
This work has been supported by the Swedish Medical Research Council (B91-39X-08705-03A) and funds of the Karolinska Institute. We acknowledge fruitful discussions with Dr Sharon Stone-Elander at the Karolinska pharmacy, Stockholm, Sweden and Dr Lars Farde, Department of Psychiatry and Psychology, Karolinska Institute, Stockholm, Sweden

7. References

Eriksson L, Holte S, Bohm C, Kesselberg M, Hovander B (1988) Automated blood sampling systems for positron emission tomography. IEEE Trans Nucl Sci 35:703-707

Farde L, Eriksson L, Blomqvist G and Halldin Chr (1989) Kinetic analysis of central D2-dopamine receptors studies by PET - a comparison to the saturation analysis. J Cereb Blood Flow Metabol 9:696-708

Greitz T.(1956) A radiological study of the brain circulation by rapid serial angiography of the carotid artery. Thesis. Acta Radiologica Suppl 140 and personal communication.

Hoffman EJ, Huang SC, Phelps ME(1979) Quantitation in positron emission tomography. 1. Effect of object size. J. Comput Assist Tomogr 3:299-308

Huang, S-H, Barrio J, Phelps M (1986) Neuroreceptor assay with positron emission tomography: Equilibrium versus dynamic approaches. J Cereb Blood Flow Metabol 6:515-521

Litton JE, Bergström M, Eriksson L, Bohm C and Blomquist G (1984) Performance study of the PC384 positron camera system for emission tomography of the brain. J. Comput Assist Tomogr 8,74-87

Litton JE, Holte S, Eriksson L.(1990) Evaluation of the Karolinska New Positron Camera System; The Scanditronix PC2048-15B. IEEE Trans Nucl Sci NS-37,743-748

Mintun MA, Raichle ME, Kilbourn MR, Wooten GF, Welch MJ (1984) A quantitative model for the in vivo assessment of drug binding sites with positron emission tomography. Ann Neurol 15:217-227

Phelps ME, Huang SC, Hoffman EJ, Selin C, Sokoloff L, Kuhl DE (1979) Tomographic measurement of local cerebral glucose metabolic rate in humans with (F-18)2-Fluoro-2-Deoxy-D-Glucose: Validation of method. Ann Neurol . 6:371-388

Rota Kops E, Herzog H, Schmidt A, Holte S, Feinendegen LE(1990) Performance characteristics of an eight-ring whole-body PET scanner J Assist Comput Tomogr.14: 437-445

Sokoloff L, Reivich M, Kennedy C, Des Rosiers MH, Patlak CS, Pettigrew KD, Sakurada O, Shinohara M(1977) The (C-14) deoxyglucose method for the measurement of local cerebral glucose utilization: Theory, procedure, and normal values in the conscious and anesthetized albino rat. J Neurochem 28:897-916

Wong DF, Gjedde A, Wagner Jr HN (1986) Quantification of neuroreceptors in the living human brain. I. Irreversible binding of ligands. J Cereb Blood Flow Metab 6:137-146.

INVESTIGATION OF THE DOPAMINE SYSTEM WITH POSITRON EMISSION TOMOGRAPHY : GENERAL ISSUES IN MODELLING

B.M. MAZOYER

ABSTRACT. A review of the major issues encountered in the modelling of PET data obtained for the investigation of the dopaminergic system is presented. Various implementations of the standard three-compartment model proposed in the literature are compared within the frame of a common set of equations and parameters. Some considerations about model validation and PET experimental protocol optimization are discussed.

1. Introduction

Besides its potential as a true diagnostic modality, Positron Emission Tomography has already emerged as an invaluable physiological and clinical research tool. The major features that make this technique so popular are threefold : - the almost unlimited possibilities of the positron emitters radiochemistry and pharmacology, - the capacity to provide absolute tissue concentration in small volumes, - the opportunity to use sophisticated mathematical modelling tools to reduce complex kinetic PET data in meaningful physiological parameters.

The most famous example of how the combination of these features can lead to a new tool for the investigation of pathophysiology is undoubtly the measurement of regional cerebral glucose metabolic rate with ^{18}F-fluoro-deoxyglucose (Phelps 1979). The way the method has been tailored for human studies is examplar : after intensive model validation in animals (Sokoloff 1977), the model has been studied in humans and its sensitivity investigated (Huang 1980). These studies led to what can now be considered as a very robust quantitative tool, and in fact a vast amount of published papers have made use of it.

J. C. Baron et al. (eds.), Brain Dopaminergic Systems: Imaging with Positron Tomography, 65–83.

It is however interesting to notice that even for this gold standard in PET methodology, there is still space available for research at the modelling level (Lammertsma 1987). Actually, modelling of PET data has emerged in the past few years as one of the most active and controversial field in PET, particularly within the frame of ligand-receptor studies (Mintun 1984). Although labelling of drugs with positron emitters has been successful very early in the history of PET (Comar 1979), modelling of ligand-receptor PET data now appears to be much more difficult than that of energy metabolic pathways data such as obtained with glucose analogs. With this respect, the measurement of dopaminergic D2 receptor density in drug naive schizophrenics has offered in the recent past a dramatic but typical example of this situation (Wong 1986c, Farde 1987, Martinot 1990). Here, different ligands, experimental protocols and model implementations have led to conflicting results and to what seemed at some point to be an endless controversy (Bice 1987, Farde 1990, Wóng 1988, Zeeberg 1988b).

In fact, the vast amount of literature on this single subject demonstrates, if needed, the hasards of modelling and the complexity of comparing data coming from different institutions. In this paper we intend to outline for readers unfamiliar with PET data modelling the major problems encountered in model building, implementation and validation with examples taken from the literature dealing with the dopamine system investigation using PET. The paper sections will follow the logical order of model development as proposed by Phelps et al (Phelps 1986) which contains the following steps :

- Tracer selection
- Derivation of a comprehensive model
- Derivation of a workable model
- Model validation
- Model application

2. Criteria for tracer selection

The first step in kinetic modelling consists in looking at which dynamic processes are under investigation. In the case of the central dopaminergic system, there are many processes that are of interest : post-synaptic receptors (D1, D2) binding kinetics, presynaptic receptor binding kinetics, autoreceptors, reuptake sites kinetics, DA synthesis, DA catabolism. Besides radiochemistry, pharmacology and radioprotection constraints, there are some criteria that positron labelled ligand must preferably fullfilled in order to be used for in vivo assays. These criteria will translate in as much hypotheses on the tracer behaviour that will help the modeller in designing his model. Obviously, these criteria are much desirable, but more often than not the true ligand properties deviate from these ideal ones.

TABLE 1 : Necessary and preferred criteria for ligands used for in vivo assays. *(adapted from Young 1986)*

1. High extraction across blood-brain barrier
2. High specificity for receptor of interest
3. If ligand binds to multiple receptor systems, receptors should be anatomically separable by spatial resolution
4. Metabolites of labelled ligand should be low and/or polar in plasma
5. Rapid clearance from blood
6. Bimolecular association and unimolecular dissociation mechanisms of receptor-ligand interaction
7. Rapid receptor-ligand association rate
8. Clearance rate from non specific sites $\leq$ clearance rate from specific sites
9. Clearance rate from non specific sites is rapid compared to radioisotope physical half-life
10. Specific activity sufficient to saturate $\leq$ 1 to 5 % of receptors
11. High affinity constant

3. Derivation of a comprehensive model

Modelling of PET data has so far almost always made use of the so-called compartmental approach in which the derivation of a comprehensive model requires an investigation about all possible fates of tracer, not only in blood and target tissue (here the dopaminergic synapses in the brain), but also in peripheral organs, especially in the ones that are possible sites of tracer catabolism and radiolabelled metabolites production.

3.1. TRACER TRANSPORT AND DELIVERY TO TISSUE

3.1.1. *Input function definition.* Although alternative strategies can be developed for practical purposes (Wong 1984, Patlak 1985) measurement of blood radioactivity components remains a necessary step in model development and can be considered as one of the most critical step in receptor-ligand modelling (Logan 1987).

Accurate measurement of the free exchangeable native ligand fraction at the blood brain barrier (BBB) level raises many questions. The first problem to be solved is to know precisely how much of the native labelled ligand is delivered at the capillary level. A large fraction of the injected ligand is usually bound to plasma protein and only a fraction (f_1, Mintun 1984) of the native radioactivity in plasma actually corresponds to the free exchangeable ligand.

Of particular importance is also the measurement of metabolites and their behaviour at the BBB level. With this respect, many of the receptor ligands so far synthetized appear to have very early release in the blood of liver produced metabolites. However, it is fortunate that these metabolites generally do not cross the BBB (Barrio 1988), and blood metabolite analysis with chromatography will ensure an accurate definition of the input function. In some cases, metabolite analysis may reveal itself unpracticable and alternative strategies have been developped to overcome this problem, such as the use of receptor free regions as input functions for receptor rich regions (Farde 1989), or the use of blockers of the ligand peripheral metabolism (Martin 1988). Incorporation of metabolite synthesis parameters in the kinetic model has also been proposed (Wong 1986a) but its validity is still a matter of controversy (Swart 1989, Wong 1989).

3.1.2. *Blood flow, permeability, and diffusion.* Ligands are delivered to brain tissue by two basic mechanisms : delivery into tissue by regional blood perfusion, and exchange between vascular and extravascular spaces across the blood brain barrier. In theory, measurements of parameters that define these two mechanisms should be performed for each experiment. However, the question of wether measurement of regional blood flow is absolutely necessary for an adequate modelling of receptor-ligand PET data is not settled yet. From the current literature, it is clear that very few experimenters (Mintun 1984, Perlmutter 1986, Perlmutter 1989) actually perform this type of investigation. The main reason for this, is the fact that blood flow and blood brain barrier transport can most of the time be confounded in a single process (in practice a single rate constant), and that it would take large flow variations to observe their influence on results (Logan 1987). One should remember, however, that simultaneous measurements of regional receptor binding parameters and perfusion might be necessary when one has some reasons to believe that perfusion may vary under high doses of the ligand, although there have not been so far any report of blood flow variation after injection of large amounts of unlabelled receptor ligands of the dopamine receptor.

3.2. FATE OF TRACER IN TISSUE

Once the various types of labelled molecules that can cross the BBB have been identified, it remains necessary to identify the kind of biophysical and biochemical pathways these molecules can enter in. Effects of molecular diffusion in the extravascular space (Zeeberg 1988c) will not be detailed because their measurements are far from reach with the PET technology.

3.2.1. *Receptor binding and enzyme kinetics.* The major process of interest is of course the binding kinetics of the ligand to its receptor. If we denote the concentration of ligand and receptor free to bind by F and R respectively, and the bound ligand concentration by B, the reaction can be described as follows :

$$F \;+\; R \;\rightleftharpoons\; B$$

$$\frac{dB}{dt} = k_{on}\;[F]\;([B_{max}] - [B])$$

where $\frac{dB}{dt}$ denotes the unidirectional rate of boud ligand formation. Here, the key point is the nonlinear bimolecular kinetics, e.g. in the fact that $\frac{dB}{dt}$ depends on the product $[F] \times [B]$. Of course, when $[B]$ is negligeable as compared to $[B_{max}]$, $\frac{dB}{dt}$ will behave as $k_{on} \times [F] \times [B_{max}]$, e.g. will follow unimolecular kinetics similar to enzyme kinetics when the substrate concentration $[F]$ is negligeable as compared to the K_m of the enzyme as shown by the following equations :

$$F \;+\; E \;\rightleftharpoons\; FE \;\rightarrow\; M \;+\; E$$

$$\frac{dM}{dt} = \frac{V_m}{K_m \;+\; [F]}\;[F]$$

The difference between the two situations is in the radiolabelled tracer kinetics : in the first case, due to the limited amount of receptor sites the presence of unlabelled ligand will modify the tracer kinetics, whereas there is usually a sufficiently large enzyme concentration to assume that the rate of substrate metabolism is constant and the same both for the labelled and the unlabelled ligand.

As for the issue of how the existence of multiple competitive sites for a given ligand would in theory modify the modelling of the PET data, it has been recently reviewed (Swart 1990) and will not be presented here.

3.2.2. *Non specific binding.* The second key question to be adressed by the modeller concerns the problem of tissue radioactivity related to non specific binding. Depending on the ligand properties, the usual attitude consists in assuming that non specific binding is negligible (Farde 1986, Farde 1989) or that there is a continuous equilibrium between the non specific compartment and the free ligand compartment (Mintun 1984, Wong 1986a, Huang 1986). This assumption will translate in the following manner : only a fraction (say f_2) of the ligand unbound to the specific receptor is free to bind to it. A very common additional assumption is to take this fraction spatially invariant. Experiments to check these hypotheses are rarely performed mostly because there are difficult to set up, and fitting for the rate constants that characterize the free / non specific exchange is equally difficult. More often than not, these quantities are thus not measured but instead are estimated on the basis of other parameters (Logan 1987, Farde 1989).

3.2.3. *Ligand metabolites in tissue.* In some cases, such as 18F-fluoro-Dopa modelling (Firnau 1988, Melega 1990), it may happen that the native ligand is metabolized in the tissue of interest. When the time constant of this process is sufficiently fast, kinetic modelling of tissue radioactivity becomes then extremely difficult, because the metabolite tissue kinetics is not separable from the native ligand tissue kinetics. In the worst possible case, tissue produced metabolite is backtransported to the blood and perturbs the blood kinetics as well. In this case, additional connstraints are needed to solve for the parameters of interest (Gjedde 1990, Yu 1990).

4. Derivation of workable models

Assuming that all previous steps have been successfully passed and that a comprehensive model has been derived, when one tries to figure out the number of compartments and parameters a realistic model of dopamine system should have, he realizes that a simple PET experiment is very unlikely to provide enough data to solve for all parameters. Figure 1 shows an already complicated but far from reality model that could be used for PET data modelling.

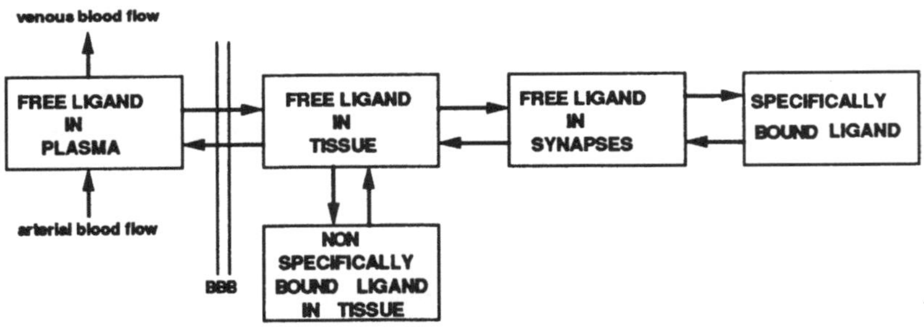

Figure 1. Comprehensive model for receptor-ligand interactions as observed with PET.

The adequacy of data and model complexity is a general issue in the modelling field, but it has been sometimes kept in the background and further comments on this issue will be given in the sixth section of the paper. To deal with this problem, there are two different attitudes : to obtain more data about the system behaviour, or to reduce the model complexity. The first approach leads to complex experimental protocol (multiple tracers, injections or measurements), while the second approach leads to simpler model and reduced number of parameters. The price to be paid in the latter approach is the difficulty to interpret the estimated parameters in meaningful biological terms and to estimate their sensitivity to deviations from assumptions that permitted the simplification of the model.

4.1. REDUCING THE NUMBER OF COMPARTMENTS

There are basically two ways of reducing the number of compartments in a model : either by asssuming that exchange rate constants between a given compartment (say NS) and others are very large (as it is hypothesized for non-specific binding for example) or that they are extremely small. In the first case, a constant equilibrium is assumed between a given compartment and another one so that only a fraction of this compartment is actually free to exchange with other compartments.The hypothesis translates in a reduction by a given factor (such as f_2) of all output rate constants. In the second case the compartment is simply neglected.

4.2 REDUCING THE NUMBER OF PARAMETERS

The second way of simplifying the model structure is to reduce the numbers of parameters to be estimated. This can be done by assigning constant values to some parameters or to some combinations of parameters. The typical case is to be found in the modelling of irreversible ligand where it is assumed that k_4 is 0. Another typical example is when it is assumed that high specific activity (SA) experiments lead to negligeable receptor occupancy, and legitimates the substitution of bimolecular kinetics by linear kinetics. As we shall see later, this will reduce the number of parameters by one, because only the product $k_{on} \times B_{max}$ can be estimated, but none of them separately. A last example can be found when the value of some combined parameters such as $f_2 \times B_{max} \times k_D$ is set to some predefined value estimated with in vitro data (Huang 1989). Again, the validity and sensitivity of these additional hypotheses should be tested inasmuch as it is possible.

4.3 THE BASIC 3 COMPARTMENT MODEL

Unless otherwise specified, we will assume in the following that we have reduced the model to the basic 3 compartment model of Figure 2 (which similar to the FDG model) that is used by a vast majority of authors as demonstrated by a survey of the litterature.

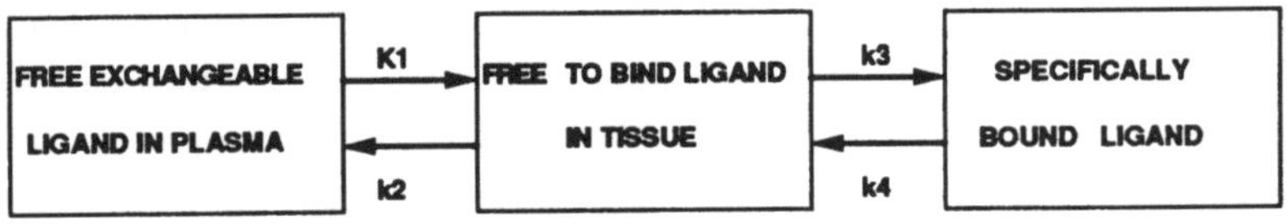

Figure 2. Workable model for receptor-ligand interactions as observed with PET.

The set of differential equations associated with this model is :

$$\frac{dC_f}{dt} = K_1 C_p - (k_2 + k_3) C_f + k_4 C_b$$

$$\frac{dC_b}{dt} = k_3 C_f - k_4 C_b$$

In these equations C_f denotes the fraction of tissue ligand free to bind to receptors, C_p the fraction of blood ligand free to cross the blood-brain barrier, and C_b the fraction of tissue ligand bound to receptors. The key point to be remembered is that, as opposed to the FDG model, the rate constant k_3 is time dependent, because of the intrinsic bimolecular kinetics of the receptor ligand interaction. In Huang's formulation (Huang 1986), k_3 is written as :

$$k_3 = k_{on} \left(B_{max} - \frac{C_b}{SA} \right) f_2$$

$$k_4 = k_{off}$$

Wong and Gjedde (Wong 1986a, Gjedde 1987) adopted a different formulation by rewriting k_3 and k_4 as :

$$k_3 = k_{on}\ B_{max}\ f_2$$

$$k_4 = k_{off}\ +\ k_{on}\ \frac{C_f}{SA}\ f_2$$

In this latter expression, k_3 is a time constant whereas it is k_4 that varies with time. The potential pitfalls of this latter formulation have been detailed by Huang (Huang 1987).

5. Model implementation

Although most of the authors in the field agree on the model structure and equation formulation, there have been many ways of adjusting this model to PET data. One of the difficulties in analyzing the literature is indeed to figure out how these different model implementations refer to each other. In this section, we tentatively compare them within the framework offered by the set of the equations previously presented. Methods are ordered with respect to the computational complexity of data to be handled, which roughly corresponds to the complexity of the experimental protocol. Comparisons of different implementations for the same ligand can be found in the literature (Bahn 1989, Farde 1989, Jovkar 1990, Logan 1990, Zeeberg 1988a) and in the next chapter of this book.

5.1. EQUILIBRIUM APPROACH

In the equilibrium approach PET data are acquired when the radioactivity has reached either a plateau or a flat peak. Two implementations of this method on two different ligands have led to similar conclusions in clinical studies (Farde 1987, Martinot 1990).

5.1.1. *The Striatum to Cerebellum ratio method.* This method has been used for brominated ligands such as spiperone and lisuride (Maziere 1985) that slowly reach equilibrium . At plateau, the previous equations become :

$$C_f = \frac{k_1}{k_2} C_p, \quad C_b = \frac{k_3}{k_4} C_f, \quad S = \frac{k_1}{k_2} \left(1 + \frac{k_3}{k_4}\right) C_p,$$

$$C = \frac{k_1}{k_2} C_p, \quad k_{on} \left(B_{max} - \frac{C_b}{SA}\right) f_2 C_f = k_{off}\, C_b$$

where S and C represent the radioactivity concentrations in the striatum and in the cerebellum respectively. The ratio of these two concentrations will write as :

$$\frac{S}{C} = 1 + \frac{k_3}{k_4} = 1 + f_2 \frac{B_{max}}{K_D}$$

The method is easy to implement and is quite to robust to the non equilibrium situation. However, it does not allow separate estimations of B_{max} and K_D.

5.1.2. *Equilibrium analysis.* This method has been designed for reversible ligands (such as Raclopride) that reach a secular equilibrium (e.g. for which B/F reaches a maximum) during the PET experiment (Farde 1986, Farde 1989). The equations ruling this type of experiment are :

$$\frac{dC_b}{dt} = 0, \quad k_{on} \left(B_{max} - \frac{C_b}{SA}\right) f_2 C_f = k_{off}\, C_b$$

$$B = \frac{C_b}{SA}, \quad F = f_2 \frac{C_f}{SA}, \quad \frac{B}{F} = \frac{B_{max} - B}{K_D}$$

In practice F is taken as the concentration in the cerebellum and B as the difference between the total radioactivity in the putamen and F. Again, the method is easy to implement and has been proved to robust to the non equilibrium conditions. With two measurements (without and with protection) separate estimations of B_{max} and K_D can be obtained.

5.2. KINETIC APPROACHES

Kinetic approaches can be divided in two categories : graphical methods for which a parameter of interest is estimated by linear regression of some function obtained by transformation of PET data, and transient analyses in which parameters are estimated by non-linear fit of a model to PET data.

5.2.1. *Graphical methods.* This method is an adaptation of the Patlak graphical analysis of uptake curves (Patlak 1983) and has been used for irreversible ligands (Wong 1986a, Coenen 1988). Denoting by C_T the total radioactivity in the region of interest (ROI) :

$$\frac{dC_f}{dt} = k_1 C_p - (k_2 + k_3)\, C_f, \quad \frac{dC_b}{dt} = k_3 C_f, \quad \frac{dC_T}{dt} = k_1 C_p - k_2 C_f,$$

which gives after integration :

$$C_T = \left(\frac{k_1 k_3}{k_2 + k_3}\right) \int_0^t C_p dt \; + \; \left(\frac{k_2}{k_2 + k_3}\right) C_f$$

In steady-state conditions :

$$C_f = V_f C_p = \frac{k_1}{k_2 + k_3}\, C_p$$

$$\frac{C_T}{C_p} = k_3 \; V_f \; \frac{\int_0^t C_p dt}{C_p} \; + \; \left(\frac{k_2}{k_2 + k_3}\right) V_f$$

With this formulation, there is a linear relationship between the tissue to plasma ratio and the integrated plasma to plasma ratio. Although it is very easy to implement, the method is based on some critical assumptions that should be checked carefully (Patlak 1983). In particular, when k_3 is large the graph slope $k_3 V_f$ is not representative of k_3 (and thus not representative of $k_{on} B_{max}$) , but instead mostly reflects k_1 e.g. tracer delivery to tissue. Other similar formulations have been proposed (Wong 1984, Patlak 1985) in which the plasma curve is replaced by a receptor free region radioactivity curve. The method has also been modified to account for experiments where it is possible to perform a second study with a competitive inhibitor such as Haldol (Wong 1986b) which allows, under some assumptions, an independent estimation of Bmax.

Another graphical analysis has been proposed for ligand with rapid washout from tissues (Logan 1990). In this approach, the ratio of the integrated radioactivity in the ROI to the ROI radioactivity at some time is plotted versus the ratio of the integrated plasma radioactivity to the ROI radioactivity at the same time. In a given region, the slope of this curve is shown to be $(k_1/k_2) \times (1 + B_{max}/K_D) + V_p$, where V_p is the blood volume. The parameter B_{max}/K_D can be estimated by comparing the slopes of the curves obtained in the receptor rich and in the receptor free regions. The method appears to be very robust and has the advantage to use early time points.

5.2.2. *Transient analysis : single injection.* In this method, the workable model presented in section 4 is fit to the dynamic PET data in order to estimate as many parameters as possible. It can be used for reversible ligands and irreversible ligands as well, but with a single injection only a combined parameter of the association kinetics such as $k_{on} \times B'_{max}$ or B'_{max}/K_D (B'_{max} is the density of available receptors) can generally be estimated. Various implementations have been proposed in the litterature that depend on the number of fit parameters and constraints.

A first implementation (Mintun 1984, Perlmutter 1986) allows the separation of blood flow (F) and permeability (PS) components by including an intravascular compartment C_1 :

$$\frac{dC_1}{dt} = \frac{F}{V_1}(C_A - C_1) + \frac{PS}{V_1}(f_2C_2 - f_1C_1)$$

$$\frac{dC_2}{dt} = \frac{PS}{V_f}(f_1C_1 - f_2C_2) - k_{on}B'_{max}f_2C_2 + k_{off}C_b$$

$$\frac{dC_b}{dt} = k_{on}B'_{max}f_2C_2 - k_{off}C_b$$

In this implementation, C_2 denotes the extravascular radioactivity not bound to specific receptors, V_2 is fixed, f_2 is taken from cerebellum, F, V_1 and f_1 from other experiments, PS, $k'_1 = k_{on}B'_{max}$ and k_{off} are the fit parameters.

As seen previously, flow and permeability are usually confounded in a single process which leads to a simpler implementation (Logan 1987) :

$$\frac{dC_2}{dt} = k_1C_p - (k_2 + k_3)\,C_2 + k_4C_b$$

$$\frac{dC_b}{dt} = k_3C_2 - k_4C_b$$

In this formulation, the blood volume is assumed constant, the four k are fit, k_1 and k_2 are combined parameters accounting for F, PS, f_1, and f_2 and $k_3 = f_2k_{on}B'_{max}$.

Although it may at first sight appear quite different, the implementation proposed by Salmon (Salmon 1990) belongs to the same category. Here, the model is further reduced by assuming rapid equilibrium between the free and bound compartments that are pooled in a single compartment (C_E). Regional values of k'_1 and k'_2 are obtained by fitting the following equation :

$$\frac{dC_E}{dt} = k'_1C_p - k'_2C_E$$

In the cerebellum region the ratio k_1'/k_2' is the usual distribution volume (V_d^{ns}), but in the receptor rich region the same ratio, V_d^s, is equal to $V_d^{ns} \times (1 + k_3/k_4)$. As a consequence, $f_2 B_{max}/K_D$ can be estimated as $V_d^s/V_d^{ns} - 1$.

Fit of bimolecular kinetics with a single injection experiment has been tried for [18F]-fluoro-ethyl-spiperone in baboons (Jovkar 1990), the five parameters $K_1, k_2, f_2 k_{on}, k_{off}$, and B_{max} being simultaneously estimated. This study clearly demonstrated the problem of single injection protocols : at low specific activity, fits did not converge, at high specific activity $f_2 k_{on}$, and B_{max} could not be reliably estimated.

5.2.3. *Transient analysis : double injection.* To solve this problem, a double injection experiment can be performed in which two different specific activities (SA1, SA2) of the ligand are injected at two different times (0, T). The goal is to obtained in a single experiment simultaneous estimation of $B_m ax$, $k_o n$ and $k_o ff$. This type of experiment has been used for ligands such as 18F-fluoro-ethyl-spiperone (Huang 1989) and 11C-Raclopride (Blomqvist 1988, Farde 1989). The previous set of equations becomes :

$$\frac{dC_{f1}}{dt} = k_1 C_{p1} - k_2 C_{f1} - k_{on} f_2 B_{max} C_{f1} + k_{off} C_{b1} + k_{on} f_2 C_{f1} \left(\frac{C_{b1}}{SA1} + \frac{C_{b2}}{SA2} \right)$$

$$\frac{dC_{b1}}{dt} = k_{on} f_2 B_{max} C_{f1} - k_{off} C_{b1} - k_{on} f_2 C_{f1} \left(\frac{C_{b1}}{SA1} + \frac{C_{b2}}{SA2} \right)$$

$$\frac{dC_{f2}}{dt} = k_1 C_{p2} - k_2 C_{f2} - k_{on} f_2 B_{max} C_{f2} + k_{off} C_{b2} + k_{on} f_2 C_{f2} \left(\frac{C_{b1}}{SA1} + \frac{C_{b2}}{SA2} \right)$$

$$\frac{dC_{b2}}{dt} = k_{on} f_2 B_{max} C_{f2} - k_{off} C_{b2} - k_{on} f_2 C_{f2} \left(\frac{C_{b1}}{SA1} + \frac{C_{b2}}{SA2} \right)$$

$$C_{p2}(t) = 0, \quad t \leq T, constrain\ K_D f_2 = 1 pmol/g$$

The classical way consists in fitting this set of equations to the entire set of PET data by non linear least-squares methods (Farde 1989, Huang 1989). There are some potential problems with this approach, namely the quality of the input function definition and the identifiability of the entire set of parameters. In particular, application of this method to ^{18}F labelled ligands requires interpolation at late times of the blood radioactivity due to the first high specific activity injection. The necessity of constraining some parameter values to some constant (Huang 1989) or within some limits (Farde 1989) demonstrates the limit of this approach and underlines the potential numerical problems of this approach that will be described in the next section.

A different formulation of these equations has been proposed for Raclopride studies (Blomqvist 1989) that rewrites C_b as a function of C_f only :

$$\frac{dC_b}{dt} + \left(k_{off} + k_{on}\frac{C_f}{SA}\right) C_b = k_{on}\ B_{max}\ C_f$$

$$C_b = \left[k_{on} B_{max} \int_0^T C_f(t)dt\right] \times exp\left(-\int_0^T \left(k_{off} + \frac{k_{on}}{SA}C_f(t)\right) dt\right)$$

The interesting point here is the linearity of the differential equation in the parameters, which allows estimation of the various parameters (an their uncertainties) on a pixel per pixel basis in a way similar to that used for FDG data (Blomqvist 1984). Solving will obviously require an estimation of C_f, for which different approaches (such as using the cerebellum region data or an enantiomer) have been tested (Farde 1989).

6. Model validation

There is in theory only one way to validate a model, that is to obtain estimates of each parameter using independent techniques. Unfortunately, there is not a single example of such validation in humans and PET experimenters must rely on indirect and incomplete validation of their models. A first approach includes comparisons of parameter values obtained in various species (see for example Farde 1985, Barrio 1989) or between vivo and in vitro experiments.

For the modeller point of view, goodness of fit and model compatibility statistics are two ways of indirect validation of models. However, the fact that tissue radioactivity model predicted values adequately fit the experimental PET data is at best a first step that allows not to reject the model. Actually, when carefully looking at goodness of fit it is not rare to find that parts of the experimental data are better fit than others, which cannot be detected by global goodness of fit statistics such as Fischer's F but rather by residual analysis (Box 1970). This kind of analysis is rarely presented (if performed) despite its informativeness.

7. Model application

Even when 'validated', a model needs an experimental design in order to be used for the analysis of human studies. By experimental design we mean the injection (labelled and unlabelled ligands) and sampling (blood and tissue) protocols. Optimization of such designs is by itself a very active field of research where, besides the model structure, it is necessary to account for the constraints inherent of human studies (pharmacology, undesirable effects, radioprotection, duration of the study) and for tomograph performances. The basic tools of experimental design optimizations are identifiability and sensitivity analysis (see Vera 1985 for a general presentation on these topics within the frame of receptor-ligand modelling), which allows comparisons between various model implementations. When comparing models and/or implementations (Farde 1989), goodness of fit statistics should be modified to account for the number of fit parameters (Akaike 1974).

7.1. IDENTIFIABILITY ANALYSIS

Identifiability analysis tries to answer some critical questions as regards the estimation of model parameters in a given model implementation. For example, a model can be validated but non identifiable because some rate constant is too low to be reliably estimated during the time course of a PET experiment in humans. Model identifiability and its application receptor PET data modelling have been presented elsewhere (Delforge 1990). Recall that in the case of non-linear models, model are structurally identifiable but this does not mean that they are numerically identifiable. In particular, it is not rare that receptor binding parameters have large values which make them hardly identifiable (e.g. without large uncertainties) given the sensitivity and sampling capability of PET machines. In fact, in addition to goodness of fit statistics and residual pattern analysis, one should always look at parameter covariance matrix (Cramer 1946) which constitutes a practical way of comparing model parameter estimates (Zeeberg 1988a, Jovkar 1990).

7.2. SENSITIVITY ANALYSIS.

In a restricted sense, sensitivity analysis is the analysis of sensitivity functions which can be viewed as how experimental errors translate in parameter uncertainties. In a wider sense, sensitivity analysis allows the investigation of the influence of the various components of the experimental design with the goal of finding the optimal set up. The optimization criterion is usually the uncertainty on the parameter of interest, here B_{max} or some others combined parameter. These studies are of particular importance because large improvements in parameter uncertainties may be obtained this way (Zeeberg 1985, Delforge 1989).

8. References

- Akaike, H. (1974) 'A new look at the statistical model identification', IEEE Trans. Automat. Contr. 19, 716-723.
- Bahn, B. B., Huang, S. C., Hawkins, R. A., Satyamurthy, N., Hoffman, J. M., Barrio, J.

R., Mazziotta, J. C., and Phelps, M. E. (1989) 'Models for in vivo kinetic interactions of dopamine-D2-neuroreceptors and 3-(2'-[18F]fluoroethyl)spiperone examined with positron emission tomography', J. Cereb. Blood Flow Metab. 9, 840-849.
- Barrio, J. R., Huang, S.C., Phelps, M. E. (1988) 'In vivo assessment of neurotransmitter biochemistry in humans', Ann. Rev. Pharmacol. Toxicol. 28, 213-230.
- Barrio, J. R., Satyamurthy, N., Huang, S.C., Keen, R., Nissenson, C. H. K., Hoffman, J. M., Ackermann, R. F., Bahn, M. M., Mazziotta, J. C., Phelps, M. E. (1989) '3-(2'-[18F]fluoroethyl)spiperone : In vivo biochemical and kinetic characterization in rodents, nonhuman primates, and humans', J. Cereb. Blood Flow Metab. 9, 830-839.
- Bice, A. N., and Zeeberg, B. R. (1987) 'Quantification of human caudate D2 dopamine receptor density with positron emission tomography : a review of the model', IEEE Trans. Med. Imag. 6, 244-248.
- Blomqvist, G., Pauli, S., Farde, L., Eriksson, L., Persson, A., and Halldin, C. (1989) 'Determination of receptor density, association - and dissociation rate constants for radioligands with PET - A comparison between the equilibrium and the kinetic approaches', in H.A.E. Schmidt and G.L. Buraggi (eds.), Nuclear Medicine Trends and Possibilities, Schattauer, Stuttgart, pp. 324-327.
- Box, G. E. P., Jenkins, G. M. (1970) 'Time series analysis, forecasting and control', Holden-Day, San Francisco.
- Coenen, H. H., Wienhard, K., Stocklin, G., Laufer, P., Hebold, I., Pawlik, G., and Heiss, W. D. (1988) 'PET measurements of D2 and S2 receptor binding of 3-N-2'-[18F]fluoroethylspip in baboon brain', Eur. J. Nucl. Med. 14, 80-87.
- Comar, D., Maziere, M., Godot, J. M., Berger, G., Soussaline, F., Menini, C., Arfel, G., Naquet, R. (1979) 'Visualisation of 11C-flunitrazepam displacement in the brain of the live baboon', Nature 280, 329-331.
- Cramer, H. (1946) 'Mathematical methods of statistics', Princeton University Press, Princeton.
- Delforge, J., Syrota, A., and Mazoyer, B. M. (1989) 'Experimental design optimisation : theory and application to estimation of receptor model parameters using dynamic positron emission tomography', Phys. Med. Biol. 34, 419-435.
- Delforge, J., Syrota, A., and Mazoyer, B. M. (1990) 'Identifiability analysis and parameter identification of an in vivo ligand-receptor model form PET data', IEEE Trans. Biomed. Eng. 37, 653-661.
- Farde, L., Ehrin, E., Eriksson, L., Greitz, T., Hall, H., Hedstrom, C.G., Litton, J. E., Sedvall, G. (1985) 'Substituted benzamides as ligands for visualization of dopamine receptor binding in the human brain by positron emission tomography', Proc. Natl. Acad. Sci. USA 82, 3863-3867.
- Farde, L., Hall, H., Ehrin, E., and Sedvall, G. (1986) 'Quantitative analysis of D2 dopamine

receptor binding in the living human brain by PET', Science 231, 258-261.
- Farde, L., Wiesel, F. A., Hall, H., Halldin, C., Stone-Elander, S., Sedvall, G. (1987) 'No D2 receptor increase in PET study of schizophrenia', Arch. Gen. Psychiatry 44, 671.
- Farde, L., Eriksson, L., Blomqvist, G., and Halldin, C. (1989) 'Kinetic analysis of central 11C-Raclopride binding to D2-dopamine receptors studied by PET - A comparison to the equilibrium analysis', J. Cereb. Blood Flow Metab. 9, 696-708.
- Farde, L., Wiesel, F. A., Stone-Elander, S., Halldin, C., Nordstrom, A. L., Hall, H., Sedvall, G. (1990) ' D2 dopamine receptors in neuroleptic- naive schizophrenic patients', Arch. Gen. Psychiatry 47, 213-219.
- Firnau, G., Sood, S., Chirakal, R., Nahmias, C., and Garnett, E. S. (1988) 'Metabolites of 6-[18F]fluoro-L-Dopa in human blood', J. Nucl. Med. 29, 363-369.
- Gjedde, A., Wong, D. F. (1987) 'Neuroreceptor assay with positron emission tomography: definition of transfer coefficients', J. Cereb. Blood Flow Metab. 7, 517-518.
- Gjedde, A., Reith, J., Kuwabara, H., Dyve, S. (1990) 'Determining Dopa decarboxylase activity in the human brain in vivo : the complete fluoro-dopa model', J. Nucl. Med. 31, 720-721.
- Huang, S. C., Phelps, M. E., Hoffman, E. J., Sideris, K., Selin, C. J., Kuhl, D. E. (1980) ' Noninvasive determination of local cerebral metabolic rate of glucose in man', Am. J. Physiol. 238, E69-E82.
- Huang, S. C., Barrio, J. R., and Phelps, M. E. (1986) 'Neuroreceptor assay with positron emission tomography : equilibrium versus dynamic approaches', J. Cereb. Blood Flow Metab. 6, 515-521.
- Huang, S. C., Barrio, J. R., Phelps, M. E. (1987) ' Nonlinearity in modelling receptor-binding ligands', J. Cereb. Blood Flow Metab. 7, 518-520.
- Huang, S. C., Bahn, M., Barrio, J. R., Hoffman, J. M., Satyamurthy, N., Hawkins, N. A., Mazziotta, J. C., and Phelps, M. E. (1989) 'A double injection technique for in vivo measurement of dopamine D2 receptor density in monkey with 3-N-2'-18F-fluoroethylspiperone and dynamic positron emission tomography', J. Cereb. Blood Flow Metab. 9, 850-858.
- Jovkar, S., Wienhard, K., Pawlik, G., and Coenen, H. H. (1990) 'The quantitative analysis of D2 dopamine receptors in baboon striatum in vivo with 3-N-2'-18Ffluoroethylspiperone using positron emission tomography', J. Cereb. Blood Flow Metab. 10, 720-726.
- Lammertsma, A. A., Brooks, D. J., Frackowiak, R. S. J., Beaney, R. P., Herold, S., Heather, J. D., Palmer, A. J., Jones, T. (1987) 'Measurement of glucose utilization with [18F]2-fluoro-2-deoxy-D-glucose : a comparison of different analytical methods', J. Cereb. Blood Flow Metab. 7, 161-172.
- Logan, J., Wolf, A. P.,Shiue, C. V., and Fowler, J. S. (1987) 'Kinetic modeling of receptor-ligand binding applied to positron emission tomographic studies with neuroleptic tracers', J. Neurochem. 48, 73-83.

- Logan, J., Fowler,J. S., Volkow, N. D., Wolf, A. P., Dewey, S. L., Schyler, D. J., MacGregor, R. R., Hitzemann, R., Bendriem, B., Gatley, S. J., and Christman, D. R. (1990) 'Graphical analysis of reversible radioligand binding from time-activity measurements applied to N-11C-methyl-(-)-Cocaine PET studies in human subjects', J. Cereb. Blood Flow Metab. 10, 740-747.

- Martin, W. R. W., Palmer, M. R., Patlak, C. S., and Calne D. B. (1898) 'Nigrostriatal function in humans studied with positron emission tomography', Ann. Neurol. 26, 535-542.

- Martinot, J.L., Preon-Magnan, P., Huret, J.D., Mazoyer, B., Baron, J.C., Boulenger J.P., Loc'h, C., Maziere, B., Caillard, V., Loo, H., Syrota, A. (1990) 'Striatal D2 dopaminergic receptors assessed with positron emission tomography and [76Br]bromospiperone in untreated schizophrenic patients', Am. J. Psychiatry 147, 44-50.

- Maziere, B., Loc'h, C., Baron, J. C., Sgouropoulos, P., Duquesnoy, N., D'Antona, R., and Cambon, H. (1985) 'In vivo quantitative imaging of dopamine receptors in human brain using positron emission tomography and [76Br]bromospiperone', Eur. J. Pharmacol. 114, 267-272.

- Melega, W. P., Luxen, A., Perlmutter, M. M., Nissenson, C. H. K., Phelps,M. E., and Barrio, J. R. (1990) 'Comparative in vivo metabolism of 6-18F-fluoro-L-Dopa and 3H-L-Dopa in rats', Biochem. Pharmacol. 39, 1853-1860.

- Mintun, M. A., Raichle, M. E., Kilbourn, M. R., Wooten, G. F., Welch, M. J. (1984) 'A quantitative model for the in vivo assessment of drug binding sites with positron emission tomography', Ann. Neurol. 15, 217-227.

- Patlak, C. S., Blasberg, R. G., and Fenstermacher, J. D. (1983) 'Graphical evaluation of blood-to-brain transfer constants from multiple-time uptake data', J. Cereb. Blood Flow Metab. 3,1-7.

- Patlak, C. S., Blasberg, R. G. (1985) 'Graphical evaluation of blood-to- brain transfer constants from multiple-time uptake data. Generalizations', J. Cereb. Blood Flow Metab. 5, 584-590.

- Perlmutter, J. S., Larson, K. B., Raichle, M. E., Markham, J., Mintun, M. A., Kilbourn, M. R., and Welch, M. J. (1986) 'Strategies for in vivo measurement of receptor binding using positron emission tomography', J. Cereb. Blood Flow Metab. 6,154-169.

- Perlmutter, J. S., Kilbourn, M. R., Welch, M. J., and Raichle, M. E. (1989) 'Non-steady-state measurement of in vivo receptor binding with positron emission tomography : "dose-response" analysis', J. Neurosci. 9, 2344-2352.

- Phelps, M. E., Huang, S.C., Hoffman, E. J., Selin, C., Sokoloff, L., Kuhl, D. E. (1979) 'Tomographic measurement of local cerebral glucose metabolic rate in humans with (F-18)2-fluoro-2-deoxy-D-glucose : validation of the method', Ann. Neurol. 6, 371-388.

- Phelps, M. E., Mazziotta J. C., Schelbert H. R. (1986) 'Positron emission tomography and autoradiography : principles and applications for the brain and heart', Raven Press,

New York.
- Salmon, E., Brooks, D. J., Lendeers, K. L., Turton, D.R., Hume, S. P., Cremer, J. E., Jones, T., and Frackowiak, R. S. J. (1990) 'A two-compartment description and kinetic procedure for measuring regional cerebral 11C-Nomifensine uptake using positron emission tomography', J. Cereb. Blood Flow Metab. 10, 307-316.
- Sokoloff, L., Reivich, M., Kennedy, C., Des Rosiers, M. H., Patlak, C. S., Pettigrew, K. D., Sakurada, O., Shinohara, M. (1977) 'The [14C]deoxyglucose method for the measurement of local cerebral glucose utilization : theory, procedure, and normal values in the conscious and anesthetized albino rat', J. Neurochem. 28, 897-916.
- Swart, J. A., and Korf, J. (1989) 'Quantification of dopamine D2 receptors by irreversible tracer binding in the living human brain : the model-dependent correction of metabolites', J. Cereb. Blood Flow Metab. 9, 906-908.
- Swart, J. A., van der Werf, J. F., Wiegman, T., Paans, A. M. J., Vaalburg, W., and Korf, J. (1990) 'In vivo binding of spiperone and N- methylspiperone to dopaminergic and serotoninergic sites in the rat brain : multiple modeling and implications for PET scanning', J. Cereb. Blood Flow Metab. 10, 297-306.
- Vera, D. R., Krohn, K. A., Scheibe, P. O., and Stadalnik, R. C. (1985) 'Identifiability analysis of an in vivo receptor-binding radiopharmacokinetic system', IEEE Trans. Biomed. Eng. 32, 312-322.
- Wong, D. F., Wagner, H. N., Dannals, R. F., Links, J. M., Frost, J. J., Ravert, H. T., Wilson, A. A., Rosenbaum, A. E., Gjedde, A., Douglass, K. H., Petronis, J. D., Folstein, M. F., Toung, J. K. T., Burns, H. D., and Kuhar, M. J. (1984) 'Effects of age on dopamine and serotonin receptors measured by positron tomography in the living human brain', Science 226, 1393-1396.
- Wong, D. F., Gjedde, A., and Wagner, H. N., Jr. (1986a) 'Quantification of neuroreceptors in the living human brain. I : irreversible binding of ligands', J. Cereb. Blood Flow Metab. 6,137-146.
- Wong, D. F., Gjedde, A., and Wagner, H. N., Jr.(1986b) 'Quantification of neuroreceptors in the living human brain. II : inhibition studies of receptor density and affinity', J Cereb Blood Flow Metab, 6:147-153.
- Wong, D. F., Wagner, H. N., Jr, Tune, L. E., Dannals, R. F., Pearlson, G. D.,Links, J. M., Tamminga, C. A., Broussolle, E. P., Ravert, H. T., Wilson, A. A., Toung, J. K. T., Malat, J., Williams, J. A., O'Tuama, L. A., Snyder, S. H.,Kuhar, M. J., Gjedde, A. (1986c) 'Positron emission tomography reveals elevated D2 dopamine receptors in drug-naive schizophrenics', Science 234:1558-1563.
- Wong, D. F., Gjedde, A., Wagner, H. N., Jr, Dannals, R. F., Links, J. M., Tune, L. E., Pearlson, G. D. (1988) 'Elevated D2 dopamine receptors in drug-naive schizophrenics : response', Science 239,790-791.

- Wong, D. F., Gjedde, A., Young, D. (1989) 'Quantification of dopamine D2 receptors by irreversible tracer binding in the living human brain : the model-dependent correction of metabolites. Reply to Swart and Korf', J. Cereb. Blood Flow Metab. 9, 908-910.
- Young, A. B., Frey, K. A., Agranoff, B. W. (1986) 'Receptor assays : in vitro and in vivo', in Phelps, M. E., Mazziotta J. C., Schelbert H. R. (eds.), 'Positron emission tomography and autoradiography : principles and applications for the brain and heart', Raven Press, New York, pp. 96.
- Yu, D. C., Huang, S. C., Barrio, J. R., Melega, W. P., Grafton, S., Mazziotta, J.C., Phelps, M. E. (1990) 'Investigation of a 6-18F-fluoro-dopa model for estimation of its kinetic parameters in human brain', J. Nucl. Med. 31, 865-866 .
- Zeeberg, B. R., Carson, R., Bacharach, S., Green, M. V., Eckelman, W. C., and Larson, S. M. (1985) 'Theoretical analysis of optimal conditions in equilibrium imaging of in vivo receptors', IEEE Trans. Nucl. Sci. 32, 1496-1502 .
- Zeeberg B. R., and Wagner, H. N., Jr. (1987) 'Analysis for three-and four-compartment models for in vivo radioligand-neuroreceptor interaction', Bull. Math. Biol. 49, 469-486 .
- Zeeberg, B. R., Gibson, R. E., and Reba, R. C. (1988a) 'Accuracy of in vivo neuroreceptor quantification by PET and review of steady-state, transient, and equilibrium models', IEEE Trans. Med. Imag. 7, 203-212.
- Zeeberg, B. R., Bibson, R. E., and Reba, R. C. (1988b) 'Elevated D2 dopamine receptors in drug-naive schizophrenics', Science 239, 789-790.
- Zeeberg, B. R., Reid, R. C., Murphy, K. A., and Reba, R. C. (1988c) 'Theoretical effects of radioligand diffusional gradients and microcospic neuroreceptor distribution in in vivo kinetic studies', Bull. Math. Biol. 50, 423-444.

MODELISATION: APPLICATION TO THE D_2 RECEPTORS

K. WIENHARD

Abstract. The graphical analysis of receptor binding allows the determination of the appropriate model configuration in the time window of the PET-measurement. Two kinds of graphical plots are applied to tissue and blood time activity data of (^{18}F)-fluoroethylspiperone an irreversibly binding and (^{11}C)-raclopride a reversibly binding D_2-receptor ligand. A comparison of the two plots allows to check whether the asymptotic ratio between tissue and plasma activity has been reached in the measured time course. For absolute quantification, however, a more detailed model analysis is needed, requiring least square fitting of the tissue time activity data to the model equations. Semi-quantitative information about receptor binding may be obtained by a simple ratio method, which can be applied quite easily to clinical routine studies.

Introduction

The aim of D_2-receptor studies with PET is not only the three-dimensional visualisation of the receptor distribution in the human brain in vivo but the absolute quantization in terms of receptor density B_{max} and affinity constant K_D. This poses several requirements on the labeled ligand, the study protocol and the model. The ligand should have a high selectivity and affinity to the D_2 receptor with low nonspecific binding. The label should have an appropriate halflife which defines the time window of the measurement, and there should be no metabolites in tissue to avoid additional problems with the modelling of the data. The procedure of the study should be simple, safe, repeatable and applicable to patients. The model should give an adequate description of the data. A ligand with slow dissociation from the receptors requires a kinetic model analysis of the dynamic tissue time activity curves. A ligand with rapid dissociation allows also an equilibrium approach. In any case, the model should be able to determine B_{max} and K_D.

Usually compartment models are used to analyze PET data. Fig. 1 shows a series of compartment models of increasing complexity together with the quantity which they describe asymptotically. Tracers or labelled metab-

J. C. Baron et al. (eds.), Brain Dopaminergic Systems: Imaging with Positron Tomography, 85–95.

olites which do not cross the blood brain barrier are still contributing to the measured tissue activity through the cerebral blood vessels. Therefore, the cerebral volume (CBV) has to be measured in a separate experiment, e.g. with labelled CO, or taken into account as an additional fit parameter in the model equations. With a tracer entering the brain tissue pool and binding there immediately and irreversibly only the transport rate K_1 into tissue can be determined. If the tracer does not bind in tissue but is clearing back into blood, then an equilibrium between tissue and blood activity will be reached asymptotically which is determined by the ratio K_1/k_2. This is the model which describes tissue with no specific receptor binding. If the tracer binds to receptors then a further compartment has to be added with rate constants k_3 and k_4. In the case of irreversible binding $k_4 = 0$ and asymptotically the accumulation rate $K_1 \cdot k_3/(k_2+k_3)$ will be reached, where k_3 represents the product of the association rate k_{on} and the density of available receptors B_{max}, $k_3 = k_{on}B_{max}$. The relative order of magnitude between k_2 and k_3 is important: if $k_3 >> k_2$ then the accumulation rate reduces to K_1 and nothing about receptor binding can be learned. With a reversibly binding tracer an equilibrium between tissue and blood activity will be reached asymptotically which is given by $K_1/k_2(1+k_3/k_4)$ where $k_3/k_4=B_{max}/K_D$.

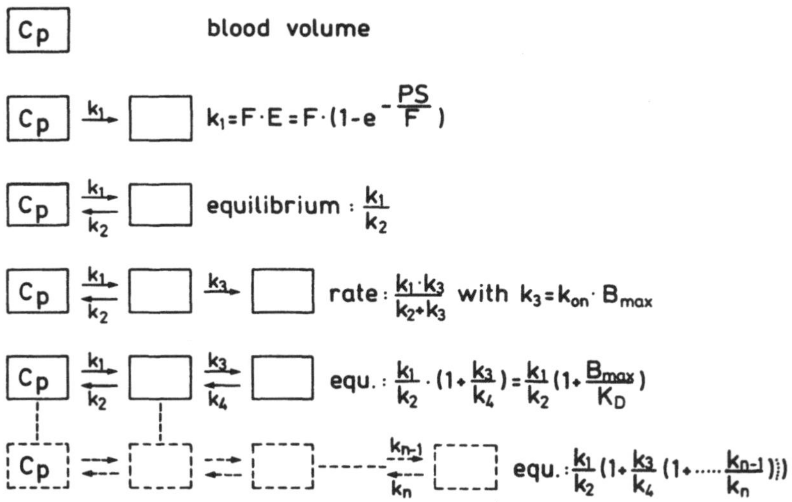

Figure 1. Compartment models of increasing complexity together with the quantity which they describe asymptotically.

One could easily go on and by adding further compartments increase the complexity of the model. However, typical PET-time activity curves (Fig. 2) do not allow to extract more than 3 to 4 model parameters unambiguously from a least squares fit to the data. If we want to decide which of the model configurations in Fig. 1 would be appropriate to fit the data in Fig. 2, we could start from the most simple models and investigate how the fit improves by adding further parameters using statistical criteria (LANDAW and DiSTEFANO 1984). This rather lengthy procedure can be simplified if we use presentations of the data which show directly the asymptotic behaviour of the different model configurations. In the following we compare tissue uptake data of (^{18}F)-fluoroethylspiperone (FESP) an irreversibly binding (COENEN et al. 1987) and (^{11}C)-raclopride a reversibly binding D_2-receptor ligand (FARDE et al. 1985) using a graphical analysis of the model configurations.

FESP - accumulation in brain tissue

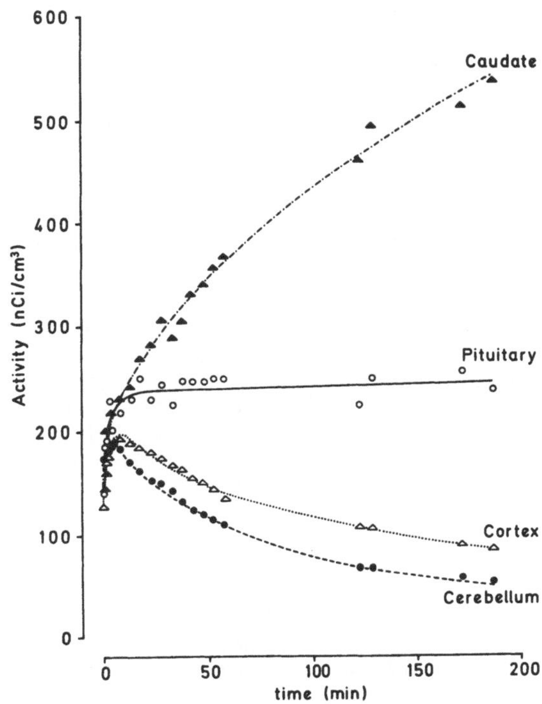

Figure 2. PET-time activity data of FESP accumulation in brain tissue over 3 hours.

Graphical analysis

A widely used graphical analysis of PET time activity data represents the Patlak-plot or Gjedde-Patlak-plot (GJEDDE et al. 1981, PATLAK et al. 1983). Here, instead of tissue activity versus time, tissue activity normalized to plasma activity is plotted versus plasma activity integrated over time and also normalized to plasma activity. This is sometimes called virtual time θ and it would be identical to real time t if plasma activity were constant in time. Such a plot (Fig. 3a) becomes linear asymptotically and in the case of a reversibly binding ligand it approaches a horizontal line with a y-axis intercept equal to the equilibrium ratio between brain and plasma activity. This ratio is equal to K_1/k_2 for a one tissue compartment model and it is equal to $K_1/k_2(1+k_3/k_4)$ for a two tissue compartment model. In the case of irreversible binding, the slope of the asymptote represents the accumulation rate of the tracer in brain tissue: $K_1k_3/(k_2+k_3)$ and the y-intercept is given by: $K_1k_2/(k_2+k_3)^2$. Another kind of graphical analysis of radioligand binding was recently applied by LOGAN et al. (1990) using a relation originally derived by PATLAK and BLASBERG (1985). In that approach, which we will name Logan-Patlak-plot in this paper, tissue activity integrated over time is plotted against the plasma-time-integral with both quantities being normalized to tissue activity (Fig. 3b). This plot also becomes linear asymptotically. For a one tissue compartment model the slope of the asymptote is given by K_1/k_2 with $1/K_1$ as x-axis and $- 1/k_2$ as y-axis intercepts. With two tissue compartments the slope is given again by the equilibrium ratio between tissue and plasma activity: $K_1/k_2(1+k_3/k_4)$, and the x-axis intercept by $1/K_1(1+k_2 \cdot k_3/(k_3+k_4)^2)$. It is interesting to look at these quantities in the case of an irreversibly binding ligand that means in the limit $k_4 \rightarrow 0$. In this case, the slope approaches infinity corresponding to an asymptotic vertical line and the x-axis intercept becomes $(k_2+k_3)/K_1\, k_3$ which is the inverse of the tissue accumulation rate of the tracer.

The two different kinds of graphical analysis contain therefore identical information but the comparison of data analyzed by both approaches may help to decide which model is appropriate in the time window of the measurement. In the above consideration, contributions from the plasma volume have been neglected for simplicity. These can in principle be measured separately and substracted from the data or they can be taken into account explicitly (PATLAK and BLASBERG 1985, LOGAN et al. 1990).

Application to D_2 receptor binding

In the following both kinds of graphical analysis are applied to typical D_2-receptor ligand PET-data. As example for an irreversibly binding ligand FESP-data (WIENHARD et al. 1990) accumulated over 3 hours and for reversible binding ^{11}C-raclopride data over 70 minutes are compared in caudate and cerebellum.*

Fig. 4a shows for FESP accumulation in caudate tissue both plots give identical results. The infinitive slope in the Logan-Patlak-plot (LP-plot) corresponds to the linear rise in the Gjedde-Patlak-plot (GP-plot) with a slope equal to the inverse of the x-axis intercept in the LP-plot. Both plots show that FESP binds irreversibly to D_2-receptors in caudate with identical values for the accumulation rate (the small difference may be due to the neglected plasma volume).

*We thank Dr. L. Eriksson and the Karolinska group for supplying us with a complete set of raclopride tissue and metabolite corrected plasma time activity data.

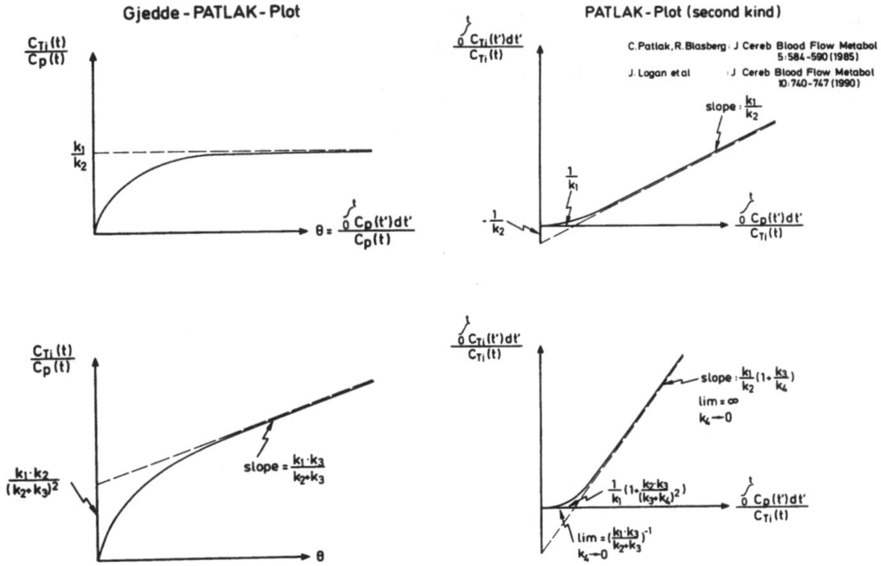

Figure 3. a. Gjedde-Patlak plots for one and two tissue compartments.
b. Logan-Patlak plots for one and two tissue compartments.

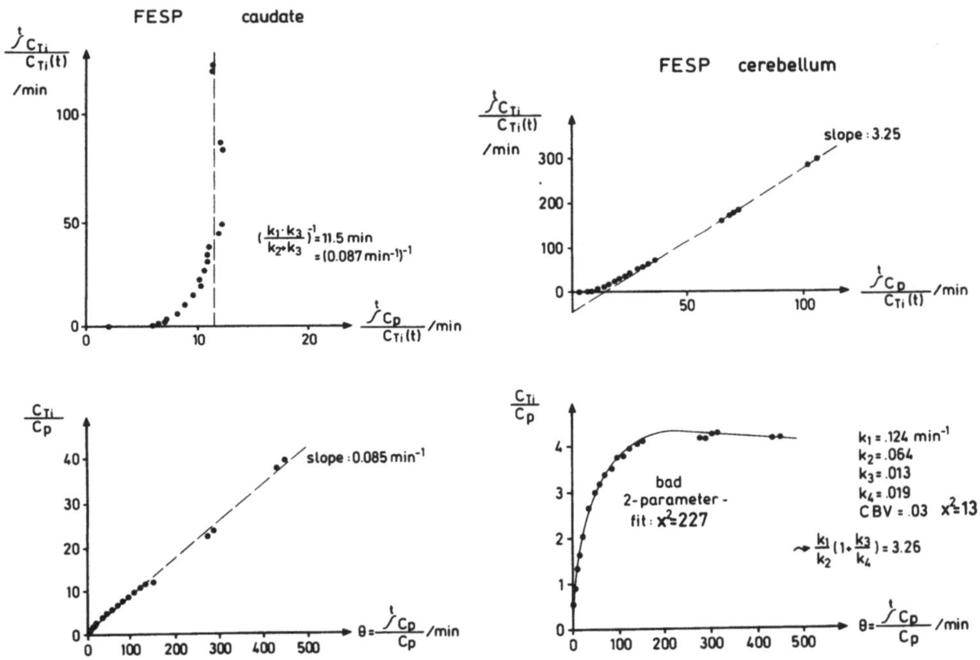

Figure 4. a. and b. Graphical analysis of FESP data in caudate and cerebellum. Upper part LP-plot, lower part GP-plot.

However, the plots of the FESP data in cerebellum in Fig. 4b seem to disagree. The LP-plot shows a linear slope of 3.25 indicating equilibrium between tissue and plasma whereas in the GP-plot this asymptotic value has not yet been reached. A fit of the time activity data with a one tissue compartment model results in a large chi-square indicating a bad approximation to the data. Adding a second tissue compartment improves the fit considerably with a value for the volume of distribution equal to the slope of the LP-plot. The need of an additional tissue compartment in the cerebellum is by no means a sufficient proof for specific binding of FESP. Tissue heterogeneity (HERHOLZ and PATLAK 1987) or other effects may simulate such an additional compartment.

The raclopride data in cerebellum (Fig. 5b) show identical results for the two plots. In the GP-plot equilibrium between tissue and plasma activity is reached after a small "overshoot" at approximately 40 min after injection with a value of the volume of distribution identical to the slope of the LP-plot. The LP-plot, however, seems to reach its asymptotic value much faster than the GP-plot as discussed by LOGAN et al. (1990). This is also evident in the plots of the raclopride data in the caudate (Fig. 5a), where the GP-plot has not yet reached its asymptotic value.

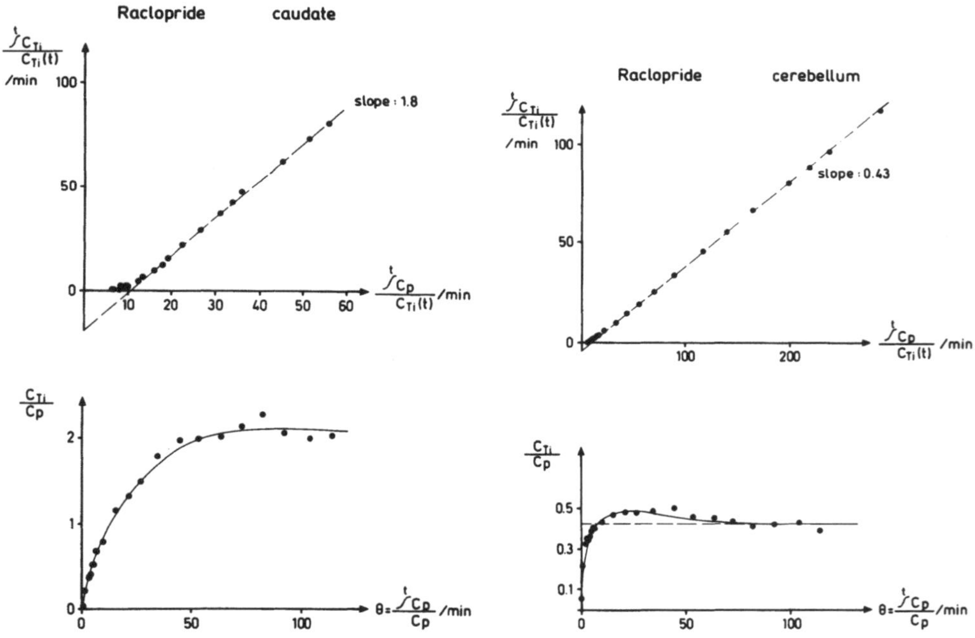

Figure 5. a and b. Graphical analysis of raclopride data in caudate and cerebellum. Upper part LP-plot, lower part GP-plot.

If one assumes that the slope in the LP-plot of the cerebellum represents K_1/k_2 and assuming that this is the same for the caudate, then the ratio of the slopes for the caudate and the cerebellum determines $k_3/k_4=B_{max}/K_d$. This simple method was successfully used in cocaine PET-studies by LOGAN et al. (1990), however it can not be applied to raclopride binding. As shown in Fig. 6, the fits to the time activity data of raclopride binding in the caudate are about equally good when cerebellar values for K_1 and k_2 are used and only k_3 and k_4 are adjusted or when all 4 rate constants are fitted. However, the derived B_{max}/K_d-values differ by almost a factor two. This is mainly due to a large difference in k_2 between cerebellum and caudate.

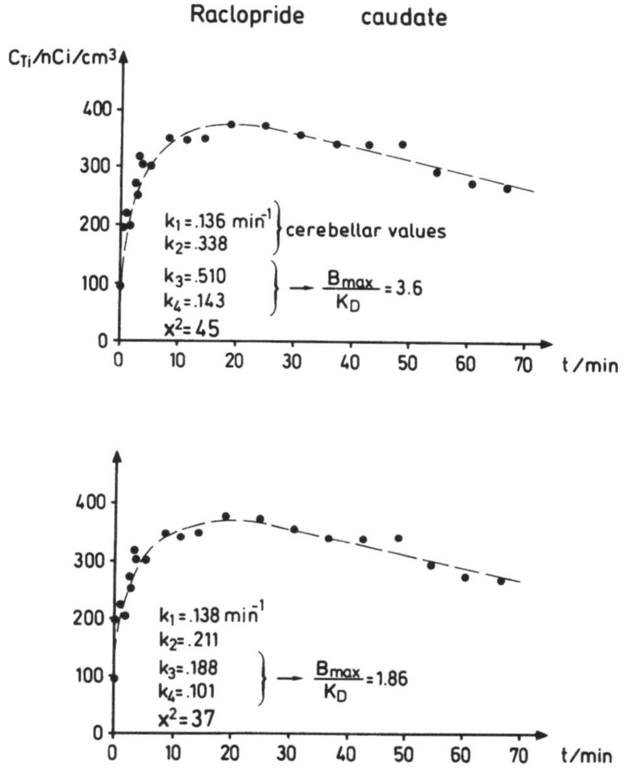

Figure 6. Comparison of fits to raclopride data in caudate. Upper part using cerebellar values for K_1 and k_2. Lower part all 4 rate constants were fitted.

From the above we can conclude that a graphical analysis of D_2-receptor binding is a simple and fast way to see qualitatively which model configuration is appropriate in the time window of the measurement. The comparison of the two Patlak-plots allows to check whether the asymptotic ratio between tissue and plasma activity has been reached in the measured time course. However, for absolute quantification of receptor binding a detailed model analysis is required. That means determination of the model parameters by least square fitting of the model equations to the time activity data. To determine B_{max} and K_D separately, studies with high and low specific activity of the tracer are necessary (HUANG et al. 1986) or the number of available binding sites must be varied by blocking with a competing ligand (WONG et al. 1986). In the case of low specific activity one has to take into account that the model equations become nonlinear (HUANG et al. 1986). For a reversibly binding ligand like ^{11}C-raclopride a much simpler equilibrium approach using a Scatchard analysis is possible (FARDE et al. 1986) which was shown to yield results similar to the kinetic analysis (FARDE et al. 1989). However, likewise at least two separate studies with differing specific activities are necessary. This large effort for the determination of B_{max} and K_D has prevented so far the broad application of these methods in clinical routine studies. Instead a simple ratio method was mostly used for clinical application (BARON et al. 1986).

Ratio method

For an irreversibly binding D_2-receptor ligand like spiperone or its analogs the ratio of activity in D_2-receptor rich tissue to that in cerebellum shows a linear rise with time after injection (Fig. 7).

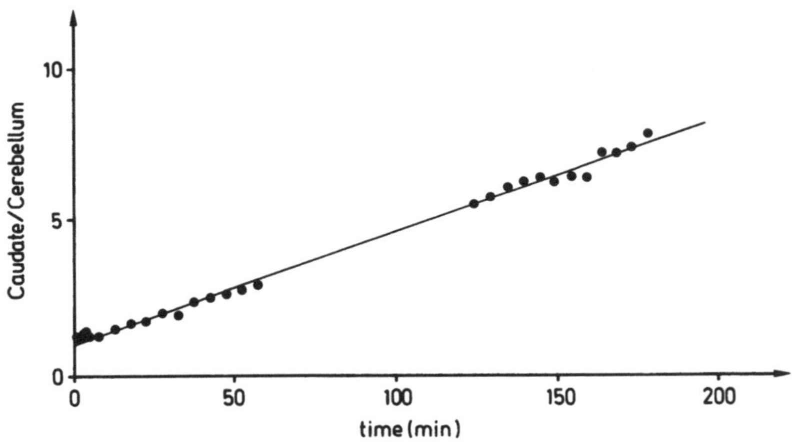

Figure 7. Caudate-to-cerebellum ratio for FESP time activity data over 3 hours.

Since at early times the ratio is close to 1, instead of the ratio at a specific time the slope of the ratio as a function of time can be used as an equivalent quantity which is independent of the time after injection. This slope has been named "ratio index". Fig. 8 shows as example the variation of the ratio index with plasma haloperidol level (WOLKIN et al. 1989). This was transformed directly to the amount of receptor occupancy as displayed in the insert of Fig. 8. The typical variation of the ratio index with receptor density is shown in Fig. 9. This curve was calculated from the model paramters of a FESP-study assuming that only k_3 changes proportional to B_{max} and that all other rate constant do not change. Because of the nonlinear dependence of the ratio index on B_{max} the sensitivity to changes in B_{max} decreases with increasing B_{max}. However, it seems strange that an almost threefold increase in B_{max} of schizophrenics was not significant in the caudate-to-cerebellum ratio (WONG et al. 1986). For reductions in B_{max} below normal values, the ratio index shows an almost linear dependence. However, one has to be careful in comparing results from different subjects, since the ratio index has also a well known age dependence (BARON et al. 1986, WIENHARD et al. 1990, WONG et al. 1984) which must be taken into account correctly. Otherwise, it does not require extended dynamic scanning and blood sampling with metabolite analysis, it is robust against exprimental errors and it is directly derived from the data without any elaborate mathematical analysis. Therefore, the ratio index is a parameter which can be easily used in a semiquantitative way in clinical routine studies.

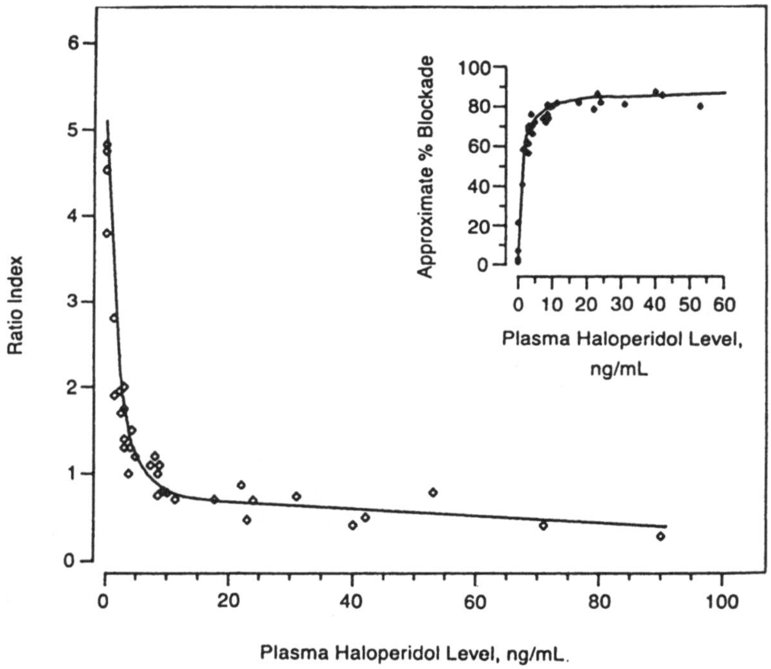

Figure 8. Relationship between plasma haloperidol level and receptor availability (ratio index) or approximate percent receptor blockade (inset). From WOLKIN et al. (1989).

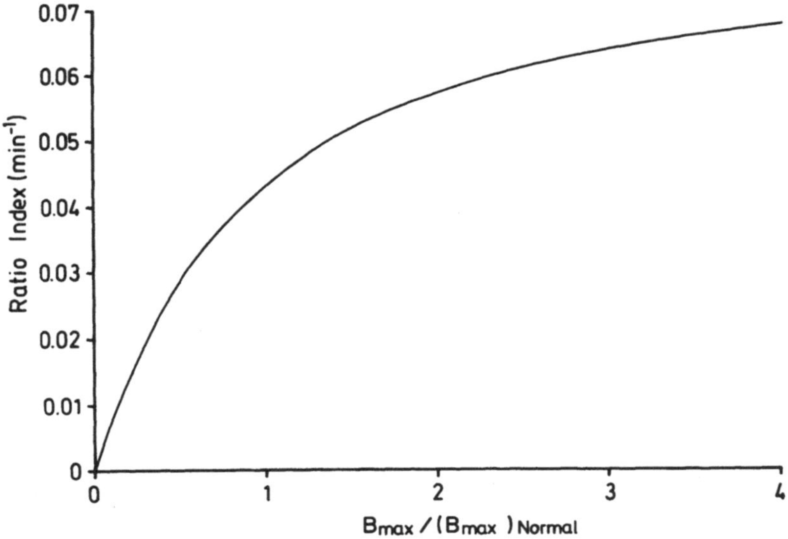

Figure 9. Theoretical dependence of the ratio index on receptor density.

References

Baron J.C., Mazière, B., Loc'h, C., Cambon, H., Sgouropoulos, P., Bonnet, A.M., and Agid, Y. (1986) Loss of striatal (^{76}Br)bromospiperone binding sites demonstrated by positron emission tomography in progressive supranuclear palsy. J. Cereb. Blood Flow Metab. 6: 131-136.

Coenen, H.H., Laufer, P., Stöcklin, G., Wienhard, K., Pawlik, G., Böcher-Schwarz, H.G., and Heiss, W.-D. (1987) 3-N-(2-(^{18}F)-fluoroethyl)-spiperone: a novel ligand for cerebral dopamine receptor studies with PET. Life Sci. 40: 81-88.

Farde, L., Ehrin, E., Eriksson, L., Greitz, T., Hall, H., Hedstrom, C.-G., Litton, J., and Sedvall, G. (1985) Substituted benzamides as ligands for visualization of dopamine receptor binding in the human brain by positron emission tomography. Proc. Natl. Acad. Sci. USA 82: 3863-3867.

Farde, L., Eriksson, L., Blomqvist, G., and Halldin, C. (1989) Kinetic analysis of central (^{11}C)raclopride binding to D_2-dopamine receptors studied by PET - A comparison to the equilibrium analysis. J. Cereb. Blood Flow Metab. 9: 696-708.

Farde, L., Hall, H., Ehrin, E., and Sedvall, G. (1986) Quantitative analysis of dopamine-D_2 receptor binding in the living human brain by positron emission tomography. Science 231: 258-261.

Gjedde, A. (1981) High- and low-affinity transport of D-glucose from blood to brain. J. Neurochem. 36: 1463-1471.
Herholz, K. and Patlak, C.S. (1987) The influence of tissue heterogeneity on results of fitting nonlinear model equations to regional tracer uptake curves: with an application to compartmental models used in positron emission tomography. J. Cereb. Blood Flow Metab. 7: 214-229.
Huang, S.-C., Barrio, J.R., and Phelps, M.E. (1986) Neuroreceptor assay with positron emission tomography: Equilibrium versus dynamic approaches. J. Cereb. Blood Flow Metab. 6: 515-521.
Landaw, E. and DiStefano, J. (1984) Multiexponential, multicompartmental, and noncompartmental modeling. II. Data analysis and statistical considerations. Am. J. Physiol. 246: R663-R677.
Logan, J., Fowler, J.S., Volkow, N.D., Wolf, A.P., Dewey, S.L., Schlyer, D.J., MacGregor, R.R., Hitzemann, R., Bendriem, B., Gatley, S.J., and Christman, D.R. (1990) Graphical analysis of reversible radioligand binding from time-activity measurements applied to (N-^{11}C-methyl)-(-)-Cocaine PET studies in human subjects. J. Cereb. Blood Flow Metab. 10: 740-747.
Patlak, C.S and Blasberg, R.G. (1985) Graphicl evaluation of blood-to-brain transfer constants from multiple-time uptake data. Generalizations. J. Cereb. Blood Flow Metab. 5: 584-590.
Patlak, C.S., Blasberg, R.G., and Fenstermacher, J.D. (1983) Graphical evaluation of blood-to-brain transfer constants from multiple-time uptake data. J. Cereb. Blood Flow Metab. 3: 1-7.
Wienhard, K., Coenen, H.H., Pawlik, G., Rudolf, J., Laufer, P., Jovkar, S., Stöcklin, G., and Heiss, W.-D. (1990) PET studies of dopamine receptor distribution using (^{18}F)fluoroethylspiperone: findings in disorders related to the dopaminergic system. J. Neural. Transm. (Gen. Sect.) 81: 195-213.
Wolkin, A., Brodie, J.D., Barouche, F., Rotrosen, J., Wolf, A., Smith, M., and Fowler, J.S. (1989) Dopamine receptor occupancy and plasma haloperidol levels. Arch. Gen. Psychiatr. 46: 482-483.
Wong, D.F., Gjedde, A., Wagner, H.N.Jr., Dannals, R.F., Douglass, K.H., Links, J.M., and Kuhar, M.J. (1986) Quantification of neuroreceptors in the living human brain. II. Inhibition studies of receptor density and affinity. J. Cereb. Blood Flow Metab. 6: 147-153.
Wong, D.F., Wagner, H.N., Dannals, R.F., Links, J.M., Frost, J.J., Ravert, H.T., Wilson, A.A., Rosenbaum, A.E., Gjedde, A., Douglass, K.H., Petronis, J.D., Folstein, M.F., Toung, J.K.T., Burns, H.D., and Kuhar, M.J. (1984) Effects of age on dopamine and serotonine receptors measured by positron emission tomography in the living human brain. Science 226: 1393-1396.
Wong, D.F., Wagner, H.N., Tune, L.E., Dannals, R.F., Pearlson, G.D., Links, J.M., Tamminga, C.A., Broussolle, E.P., Ravert, H.T., Wilson, A.A., Young, T.K., Malat, J., Williams, J.A., O'Tuama, L.A., Snyder, S.H., Kuhar, M.J., and Gjedde, A. (1986) Positron emission tomography reveals elevated D_2 dopamine receptors in drug-naive schizophrenics. Science 234: 1558-1563.

[18F]FLUORODOPA UPTAKE IN BRAIN

K.L. Leenders

ABSTRACT. In this chapter the tracer [18F]Fluoro-L-3,4-dihydroxyphenylalanine is reviewed. Particular attention is paid to pharmacokinetic issues and the problems concerning interpretation of the signal measured from the brain by PET.

1. Introduction

Fluoro-L-3,4-dihydroxyphenylalanine (FDOPA) can be labelled with fluorine-18 and used as a radiotracer in brain PET studies to investigate the dopaminergic nigrostriatal neuronal system. Particularly the decarboxylase activity of the nerve terminals projecting from the substantia nigra into the striatum can be traced with this PET method, although with the newest generation of PET tomographs also in brain regions other than the striatum specific uptake can be identified. Patients with Parkinson's disease (Leenders et al.,1986a; 1990 and others), but also other movement disorders and the effect of tracer uptake by normal ageing (Sawle et al.,1990) have been investigated.
Notwithstanding preliminary successes there are a number of methodological limitations in the application of radiolabelled FDOPA, which are to be considered. Some of these have been experimentally addressed and will be discussed below.

2. Fate of Tracer

After intravenous administration of radiolabelled FDOPA ([F18]-FDOPA) the tracer's activity in the blood can be followed by taking samples from the arterial blood. This allows one to determine the tracer input function to the tissues.
In Figure 1 the main metabolic fate of FDOPA in blood and brain tissue is schematically drawn. The metabolic pathway is qualitatively similar if not identical to exogenous L-DOPA (Firnau etal.,1986,1988; Cumming et al.,1987a,1988; Melega et al.,1990b),although at several steps there are quantitative differences in transformation or transportation.

J. C. Baron et al. (eds.), Brain Dopaminergic Systems: Imaging with Positron Tomography, 97–110.

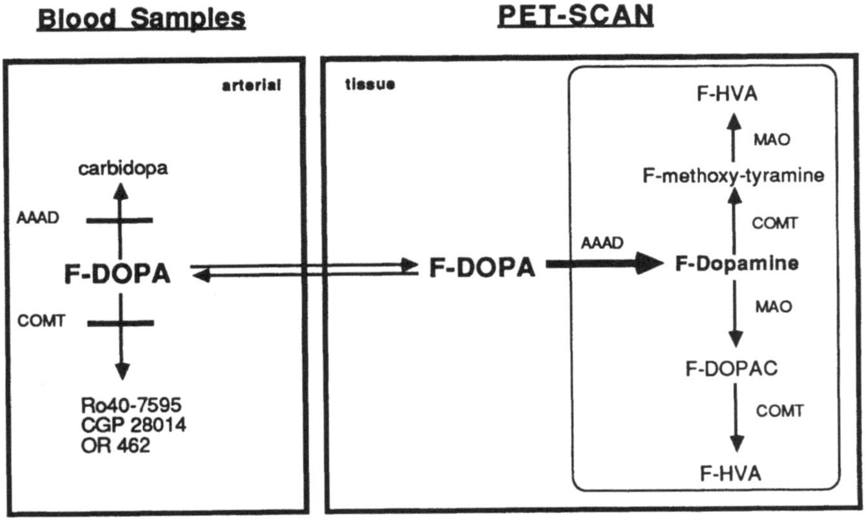

Figure 1. Schematic diagramm of fluorodopa metabolism in blood and "brain" tissue under ideal peripheral inhibitory circumstances.

2.1. PERIPHERAL METABOLISM

2.1.1. *Decarboxylation*

Decarboxylation of exogenous L-DOPA or L-FDOPA by the enzyme aromatic amino acid decarboxylase (AAAD, EC 4.1.1.26) is a major metabolic transformation resul–ting in (fluoro)dopamine (FDA) formation. The position of F-18 at the 6 position on the aromatic ring results in a Km for AAAD, that is within the range published for L-DOPA (Cumming et al.,1988). In contrast, 2-[18F]-L-FDOPA was not decarboxylated in rat striatum. Since amines do not readily pass the blood-brain barrier, peripheral decarboxylation reduces FDOPA tracer availability in the blood plasma and necessitates determination of radiolabelled FDOPA metabolic products in order to obtain a correct FDOPA input function.

When peripheral decarboxylation is prevented by sufficient carbidopa pretreatment in man and monkey, only two radiolabelled products are determined by HPLC in the plasma after administration of 6-[18F]FDOPA (Boyes et al.,1986; Melega et al.,1990; and others). However, blocking of decarboxylation increased the alternative metabolic pathway, namely the 3-O-methylation, while in man for 30 min FDOPA levels were significantly increased. Fluorodopamine (FDA) and fluorodihydroxyphenylacetic acid (FDOPAC) were not detected and fluorodopamine sulfate and fluoro-homovanillic acid concentrations were decreased (Melega et al.,1990). The same investigators found that in rat carbidopa pretreatment increased FDOPA availability to the brain and resulted in greater selective FDA accumulation in striatum.

In Figure 2 examples of time-activity curves are given of 6-[18F]-L-FDOPA PET scans performed in a healthy volunteer without and with oral pretreatment with 150 mg carbidopa. The total activity measured both in striatal and in non-striatal regions of interest is increased when carbidopa is given as pretreatment. On average in 5 subjects 30% increase of activity was found.

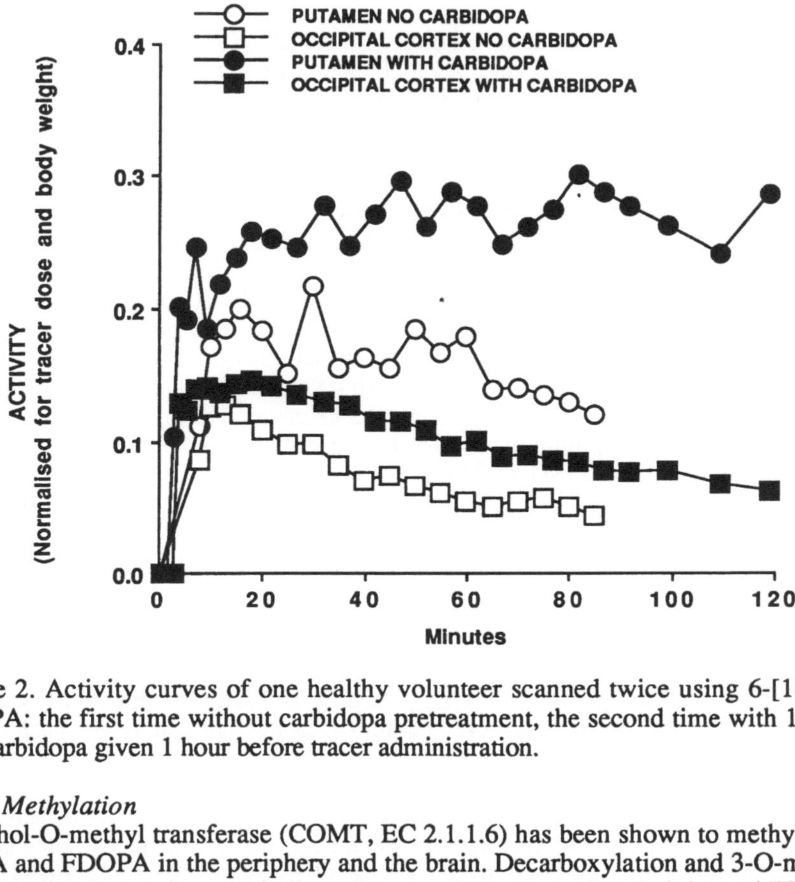

Figure 2. Activity curves of one healthy volunteer scanned twice using 6-[18F]-L-FDOPA: the first time without carbidopa pretreatment, the second time with 150 mg oral carbidopa given 1 hour before tracer administration.

2.1.2. *Methylation*

Catechol-O-methyl transferase (COMT, EC 2.1.1.6) has been shown to methylate L-DOPA and FDOPA in the periphery and the brain. Decarboxylation and 3-O-methylation are the two major metabolic pathways of exogenously administered FDOPA. This was already shown by Horne and colleagues (1984) using [3H]-L-DOPA in rats. As mentioned above the methylation products of FDOPA in plasma increased in humans 45 to 65% when decarboxylation was effectively blocked (Melega et al., 1990a). Apart from contributing to the plasma radioactivity signal and thus confounding the arterial input function, the methylated product of [18F]FDOPA does enter the brain similarly as FDOPA and add to the background signal. Reith and colleagues (1990) found the permeability of 3-O-methyl-FDOPA in rats to be twice that of FDOPA.

To minimize the radiolabelled methylation product, the 6-[18F]-L-FDOPA isomer (rather than the 2- or 5-isomer) has been selected as tracer of choice. 6-FDOPA has a low affinity and low Vmax for COMT (Creveling and Kirk,1985). Firnau and colleagues (1986) report that 5-[18F]FDOPA is methylated four times faster than L-DOPA. In contrast 6-FDOPA is O-methylated four times less than L-DOPA. 2-FDOPA is methylated twice faster than 6-FDOPA (Cumming et al., 1988).

Another approach is to add a COMT inhibitor as pretreatment, in addition to carbidopa before [18F]FDOPA administration. Until recently no COMT inhibitors for human use did exist, but now several compounds are available on an experimental basis for such an aim. Attempts have recently been undertaken to investigate [18F]FDOPA uptake in combination with a COMT inhibitor and carbidopa. One study used 6-[18F]-L-FDOPA and the COMT inhibitor U-0521 in rats pretreated with carbidopa (Cumming et al.,1987b).

With carbidopa, but without COMT inhibitor, 3-O-methylated FDOPA was the only metabolic product in cortex and cerebellum. When U-0521 was added a small lasting decrease of methylated product was found. In striatum a large lasting reduction of methylated FDOPA was found, but a 50% increase of FDA and 40% increase of FDOPAC was also noticed. The authors note that the dose used was considerably less than required to inhibit COMT fully. It is obvious that the correct dosages of the new COMT inhibitors in combination with the decarboxylation blockers need to be worked out before a reliable balance of peripheral metabolite prevention can be assumed, particularly since the COMT inhibitors seem to have rather short half lives of activity. It was found that adding a COMT inhibitor to a benseraside pretreatment scheme in a FDOPA PET study resulted in a larger availability of benseraside in the plasma and therefore in an increased permeability of this decarboxylation inhibitor into the brain which in turn resulted in reduced specific uptake in striatum (Tedroff et al., personal communication).

2.2. BBB TRANSPORT

Amino acids are taken up into the brain by specific and saturable transport systems. Each transport system will take up several amino acids in competition with each other. The L(leucine) transport system is the predominant neutral amino acid transport system and both L-DOPA and 3-O-methyldopa compete for it (Wade and Katzman, 1975). The transport is non-energy requiring, sodium independent and also called facilitated diffusion (as determined by Michaelis-Menten kinetics). In accordance with the notion that the large neutral amino acid transport is reversible, Garnett and colleagues (1980) found that 80% of the FDOPA extracted was returned to the blood. However, the concept of symmetrical transport of amino acids across the blood-brain barrier was recently challenged (Knudsen et al.,1990).

For the blood-brain transport it is important at which position on the ring the F18 label is: 2-[18F]-L-FDOPA passes the barrier less readily than the 6-isomer (Cumming et al.,1988). The transport of 6-[18F]FDOPA into brain occurs at the same rate as DOPA (Reith et al., 1990). This seems also true for the 5-isomer (Garnett et al.,1980).

Using PET and L-[18F]FDOPA in a healthy volunteer global cerebral competition with normal amino acids could be demonstrated (Leenders et al., 1986b). In that study a moderately large plasma concentration of amino acids was applied to demonstrate a clearcut blocking of FDOPA uptake into brain. Also everyday changes of plasma amino acid levels seem to have a systematic influence on the K1 value of [18F]FDOPA when applying kinetic tracer models (Melega, personal communication). When precise measurements of FDOPA uptake are needed, then it may be necessary to determine plasma amino acids in the subject under study, or apply a standard fasting protocol.

2.3. CEREBRAL METABOLISM

The fate of 6-[18F]-L-FDOPA in brain tissue is nowadays fairly well known. Melega and colleagues (1990b) compared the biochemistry of this tracer in a double-label experiment with that of [3H]L-DOPA in rat brain. After carbidopa pretreatment the major metabolites in the periphery were 3-O-methyl-DOPA and 3-O-methyl-fluoro-DOPA. The methylated metabolites entered striatum and cerebellum significantly and uniformly. The dopamines were the major metabolites (approximately half of the activity) formed in the striatum itself, whereas the rest of the measured activity mainly derived from the methylated products of peripheral origin. In the cerebellum only the dopa tracers themselves and their 3-O-methylated products were found (at 60 minutes 90% of cerebellar 18-F activity related to the 3-O-methylated product). An important clue, that after exogenous (F)DOPA administration the methylated products in brain tissue come from the periphery, can be derived from the stable ratio of methylated products in striatum to cerebellum over time, notwithstanding the actually changing values in both brain regions. A similar finding in rats using [14C]-L-DOPA has been presented (Horne et al.,1984).

In striatal regions exogenous DOPA is rapidly decarboxylated in the nerve terminals of the nigrostriatal dopaminergic system (Lloyd et al.,980; Horne et al.,1984; Hefti et al.,1984; Brannan et al.,1989; and others). For radiolabelled FDOPA the same has now been demonstrated in rats (Melega et al.,1990b) and primates (Firnau et al., 1987). The Km of 6-L-FDOPA (100 μM) for AAAD has been shown to be in the range of DOPA (Cumming et al.,1988). In fact, the kinetic constants determined for 6-L-FDOPA suggest that this substance is almost as good as substrate for AAAD as L-DOPA.

Another interesting point in the metabolic fate of FDOPA is the turnover pools into which this substance may enter. The findings of Melega and colleagues (1990b) point to a slow central oxidation since the concentrations of fluorinated or tritiated DOPAC and HVA are low. Also the level of formed FDA and DA did hardly decrease during the period of study. Endogenous striatal dopamine has an overall half-life of approximately 2 hours. These authors suggest that exogenous FDOPA enters a slow turnover rate functional pool. The notion of at least two dopamine pools in striatal dopaminergic nerve terminals, a larger but slower one (half life 2 hours) and a smaller but more rapid one (half life 9 min), has been present for some time (Doller and Connor,1980; and others). On the other hand Reith and colleagues (1990) argue that in rat brain FDOPA enters only for 1% the larger pool while most of the in striatum synthesised fluorodopamine is suggested to be metabolised rapidly without entering the large pool. The latter findings are based on kinetic calculations (see below) yielding a mean value for k3 (rate constant for FDOPA decarboxylation) of 0.010 min^{-1}. According to biochemical values from the literature (Vmax and Km of L-DOPA for AAAD) the authors predicted a value of around 1 min^{-1} (Firnau et al., 1986, however, calculate a value of 0.11). Of interest is that the k3 values calculated using 6-[18F]-L-FDOPA PET scans in healthy volunteers were equally around 0.010 min^{-1} (cerebellum as reference) (Leenders et al.,1990) in accordance with the outcome of the kinetic calculations of Reith and colleagues (1990).

Clearly, direct comparison of biochemical and kinetic data is necessary to solve above mentioned controversy, or to come to a better understanding into which functional sub-pool exogenous L-DOPA or L-FDOPA enters.
Notwithstanding yet unsolved quantitative relations, F-dopamine mimics central dopamine metabolism remarkably well. No evidence exists to show that F-dopamine synthesis from *exogenous* FDOPA is related to *endogenous* dopamine synthesis. The erroneous but often heard opinion that FDOPA tracer uptake in striatum relates to endogenous dopamine concentration is unfortunately a misleading concept.

3. Quantification

3.1. RATIO'S

Ratios calculated from some part of the time-activity curve of the target region of interest (ROI) to a reference ROI is a very simple method and provides within certain limits a robust estimate of specific tracer uptake. Cumming and colleagues (1988) found that "The ratio of total radioactivity between striatum and other brain regions is related to the decarboxylation of radiolabelled tracer and the relative persistence of the decarboxylated derivatives in the striatum" in their rat studies using 6-[18F]-L-FDOPA. Also Melega and co-authors (1990) found in rat brain tissue a parallel increase over time in the ratio of total activity in striatum to cerebellum after injection of the tracers [3H]DOPA and [18F}FDOPA. In some situations such an index can already be sufficient to provide limited biological or pathophysiological answers (Leenders et al.,1986a).

3.2 GRAPHICAL EVALUATION OF BLOOD-TO-BRAIN TRANSFER

Patlak and colleagues (1983,1985) developed a theoretical model which within certain limitations describes blood-to-brain exchange of tracer substances. The data processing requirements are rather simple: the calculation of a ratio between target ROI and reference plotted against normalised time (also called "stretched" or "equivalent" time). This "Multiple Time Graphical Analysis (MTGA)" will yield a curve that eventually will become linear if basic assumptions are met. One of these assumptions is accurate determination of a single input and the existence of a final "irreversible" kinetic compartment in the target tissue. However, generalisations can be allowed for (Patlak et al.,1985) and the system appears to be quite robust when applied to [18F]FDOPA tracer measurements. The model description is not based on the mathematical terms of a particular compartmental model, but the slope (= net influx constant or K_i) and intercept (= steady state volume of distribution) of the linear part of the MTGA plot can be expressed in the rate constants of a three compartment model.
In Figure 3 it is shown, that for 6-[18F]-L-FDOPA the arterial plasma input activity can be transformed to yield units of time which is directly proportional to real time. An actual point in time of the arterial curve, for instance 50 minutes, is "stretched" to almost 100 minutes in the example given. Against this "linearised" input the ratio of target ROI to reference is plotted. In figure 4 several examples are given. It can be seen that the regression line of the putamen/plasma ratio has a clearly bigger upward slope than that of the cerebellum. The latter one often even shows a slight negative slope.

Most likely this is due to radiolabelled metabolite formation in the blood which was not accounted for in the examples given (although carbidopa 150 mg was given orally).
When other brain regions are taken as reference, e.g. cerebellum then a non-dopaminergic brain region like occipital cortex will show a vitually horizontal course. Using an intracerebral reference the slopes of the regression lines will always be larger than when arterial plasma is the reference, but the relationships between the slope values remain the same (Leenders et al.,1990). The slope may then directly reflect k3, if k3 is much smaller than k2 (Patlak et al.,1985). This condition is however hardly fulfilled since for 6-[18F]-L-FDOPA k2 is only approximately 8 times bigger than k3 (Keith et al.,1990).
When considering the fact that in cerebellum after tracer injection only the tracer itself and its methylated form are present, it is possible to subtract the cerebellar value from the total striatal value to be left with the specifically trapped FDOPA signal. When using this value in the plotting of the MTGA graph with metabolite corrected plasma activity a better linearisation can be obtained which also starts earlier in time (Sawle et al.,1990).

3.3. KINETIC MODELLING

Since after transportation of 6-[18F]-L-FDOPA from the blood into brain the first irreversible metabolic conversion is the decarboxylation step after which the product is essentially trapped for the duration of the PET measurement, a three compartmental model and its formal mathematical solution does apply. This entails curve fitting routines relying on accurate plasma input and tissue response data sets. In general it seems preferable for the calculation of transfer constants if the number of possible kinetic compartments can be reliably reduced, if - as is usually the case in PET studies - only two data sets are available.
As will be clear from the previous paragraphs of this chapter, an accurate plasma input function of 6-[18F]-L-FDOPA can be obtained only if in the periphery, apart from the decarboxylation, also the methylation of the tracer can effectively be blocked. It needs to be confirmed experimentally that dual peripheral inhibition indeed yields a sufficiently pure arterial plasma input curve. It remains to be seen whether a COMT inhibitor which also blocks COMT in the brain is preferable to an inhibitor which is active only in the periphery, since it has been shown, that the methylated tracer product detected in the brain is most likely stemming from the periphery (see above).
Because of the slow accumulation of specific intrastriatal signal after 6-[18F]-L-FDOPA administration a formal kinetic analysis is hampered by poor counting statistics. This might be less of a problem with newer PET scanners designed to provide a higher signal to noise for low counting rate situations like after 6-[18F]-L-FDOPA administration.

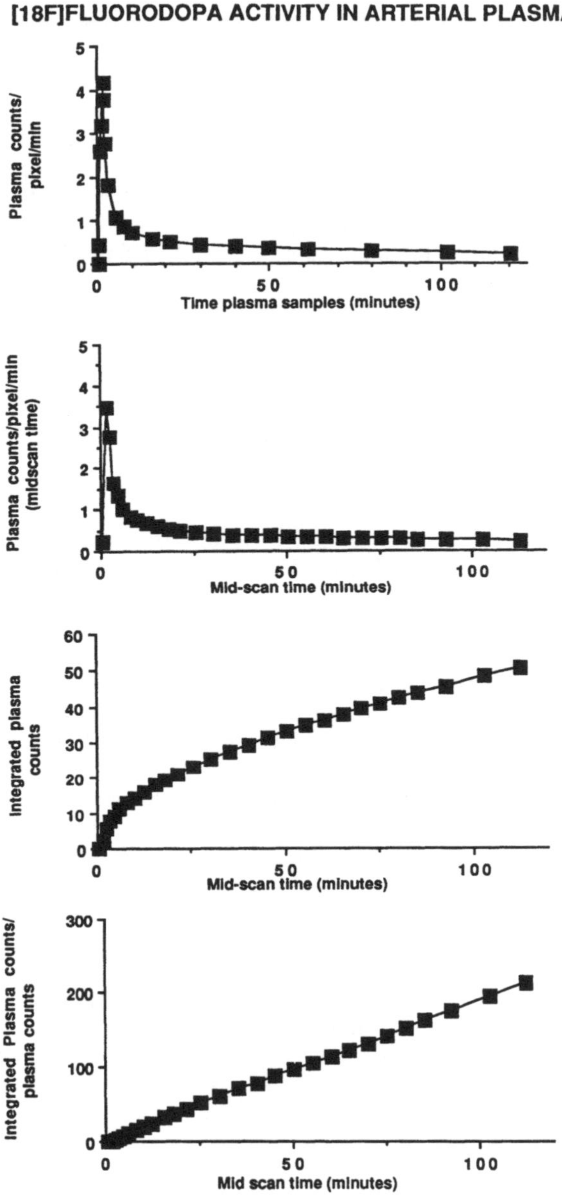

Figure 3. Radioactivity curve in arterial plasma samples after 6-[18F]-L-fluorodopa administration in a healthy volunteer. The same data are used in all four panels to illustrate the transformation of the input curve (top panel) into a straigth line (bottom panel) directly proportional to real time.

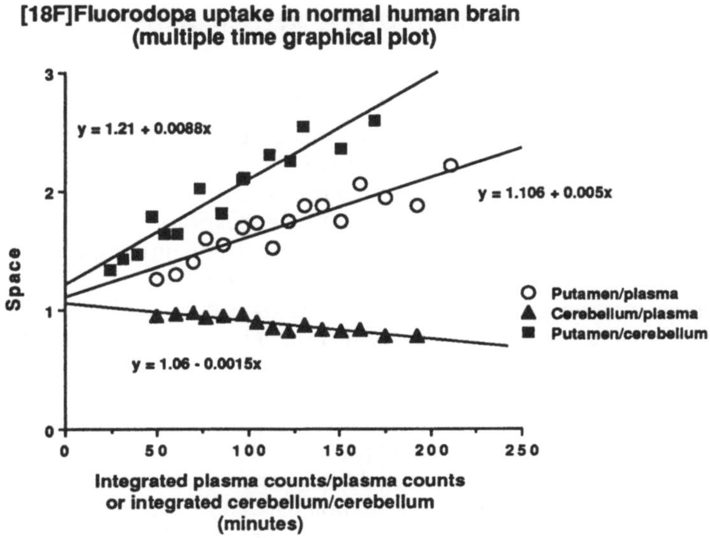

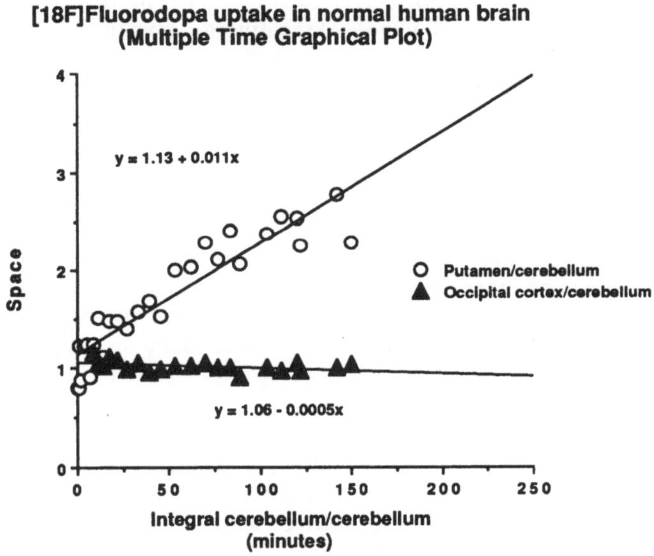

Figure 4. Several examples of multiple time graphical analysis (MTGA) plots. For explanation see text. In the upper plot the putamen of the same subject is plotted twice, once with arterial plasma as reference and once with cerebellum value as reference.

4. Interpretation of [18F]FDOPA derived Activity

The considerations summarised in paragraph 2.3 particularly must lead to the conclusion, that in striatum the fraction of 6-[18F]-L-FDOPA derived radioactivity which is calculated as measured with PET to be specifically processed in the tissue, reflects directly tracer decarboxylation and subsequent retention of the decarboxylation products (mainly 6-[18F]FDA). On the basis of several experimental findings listed above the one-way metabolic pathway of FDOPA appears to result in a better "chemical resolution" - within the special neurobiological dopaminergic organisation of the striatum - than theoretically might seem to be the case.
It has to be stressed again that 6-[18F]-L-FDOPA does not measure the endogenous dopamine pool or metabolic pathway thereof. Tracer kinetically there is no apparent equilibrating activity between the endogenous dopamine pathway and 6-[18F]-L-FDOPA. The tracer mimics exogenous L-dopa uptake. It remains to be solved into which subtype of kinetic pool exogenous L-dopa enters and what significance this has, on the one hand, for the interpretation of 6-[18F]-L-FDOPA tracer kinetics, and, on the other hand, for our understanding of tissue dopaminergic biochemistry.
In Parkinson's disease the decarboxylation capacity in striatum, particularly caudate nucleus, may be retained to a considerable extent, whereas the endogenous dopamine concentration may be more markedly decreased. This has recently been discussed in detail (Leenders et al.,1990). In Parkinson's disease the decarboxylation capacity seems to reflect more the density of remaining nigrostriatal nerve terminals rather than endogenous dopamine concentration. If in other "basal ganglia diseases" the primary pathological insult is not the endogenous dopaminergic production, but the dopaminergic cell (or nerve terminal) itself, then in such circumstances it might be anticipated that nerve terminal loss correlates with decreases in AAAD and endogenous dopamine concentration.Still, the tracer 6-[18F]-L-FDOPA would not in that case directly measure endogenous dopamine content.

5. Recommendations

From the foregoing several recommendations concerning PET measurements using 6-[18F]-L-FDOPA can be made. They should in no way be regarded as comprehensive or as decisive, since new findings and technical developments may most likely add or modify our concept of 6-[18F]-L-FDOPA uptake into brain.

5.1. DIET AND DRUGS

Since large changes in plasma amino-acid levels do influence 6-[18F]-L-FDOPA brain uptake it is advisable to take this into account. If simple indicators like ratio's for specific tracer uptake are used, it may suffice to make sure that subjects are always scanned in the same fasting condition. If more rigorous and subtle calculation protocols are employed to estimate kinetic rate constants, then accurate determination of aminoacids in blood may prove necessary to account for small changes in plasma level. However, this has not been demonstrated yet in a convincing way.

The same reasoning applies to levodopa and 3-O-methyl-dopa levels. When simple indicators are used an over-night withholding of levodopa drug therapy may suffice. It has been argued that usually the plasma levels of levodopa and 3-O-methyl-dopa are not high enough to effect competition of transport at the blood-to-brain barrier. This equally has not been settled satisfactorily in man using PET.

5.2. PRETREATMENT

Carbidopa as peripheral decarboxylation inhibitor has certainly proven its value in cleaning up 6-[18F]-L-FDOPA uptake kinetics. The author administers 150 mg one hour before tracer administration, but different protocols may result in similar peripheral decarboxylation blockade. The use of COMT inhibitors is currently under investigation in several groups. It will be most likely that soon recommendations can be published concerning the addition of methylation inhibition.

5.3. SCAN PROTOCOL

The scan protocol depends heavily on which calculation method is going to be employed to determine specific tracer uptake. When only ratio's between striatal and non-dopaminergic regions are determined, no measurement of blood activity nor dynamic scan measurements are necessary. One static measurement between 1 and 1.5 hour would then suffice. With increasing demands on accuracy and subtlety of the applied tracer model more sophisticated measurement protocols are mandatory as outlined above. It is recommended to measure in any event the dynamic tracer uptake in the brain since this also will allow - apart from calculation of simple ratio's - to apply the graphical plotting method with a non-dopaminergic brain region as reference. This will provide a rough estimate of the kinetic constant k3 when tracer processing is viewed from a 3-compartmental system. For research purposes the aim should be to design a protocol as extensive as possible, including elaborate plasma measurements. The duration of the measurement is not fixed, but has commonly been until 1.5 hour after tracer application. This has been found empirically, since from 30 to 90 minutes after tracer administration the graphical plot method using plasma as reference proved to be "linear" and since in that time interval a sufficient number of scan time frames can be collected to indeed establish a rough linearity of the curve.

5.4. CALCULATION METHOD OF CHOICE

In principal a dynamic rigorous kinetic approach of the measured tracer uptake is recommended. However, the necessary determination of radiolabelled metabolites in plasma may pose unsurmountable logistical barriers in many laboratories. This problem might in the future be solved when sufficient dual peripheral inhibition of metabolite formation can be achieved by pretreatment of an appropriate combination of carbidopa and COMT inhibitor. The resulting total arterial plasma radioactivity would then derive from 6-[18F]-L-FDOPA only, simplifying the measurement protocol significantly.

In the absence of an accurate plasma input curve the best method to apply is probably the simple but robust "multiple time graphical plotting" technique (see paragraph 3.2) using non-dopaminergic brain tissue as reference. The slope of the regression line through the linear part of the curve theoretically yields an estimate of k3, direcly reflecting the rate of specific tracer processing, i.e. 6-[18F]-L-FDOPA decarboxylation. The accuracy of this estimate needs further validation however.

References

Boyes, R. E., Cumming, P., Martin, W.R.W. and McGeer, E. G. (1986) "Determination of plasma [^{18}F]-6-fluorodopa during positron emission tomography: elimination and metabolism in carbidopa trated subjects", Life Sciences 39, 2243-2252.

Brannan., T., Knott, P., Faufmann, H., Leung, L. and Yahr., M. (1989) "Intracerebral dialysis monitoring of striatal dopamine release and metabolism in response to L-DOPA", J. Neural Transmission 75,149-157.

Creveling, C. R. and Kirk, K. L. (1985) "The effect of ring-fluorination on the rate of O-methylation of dihydroxyphenylalanine (dopa) by catechol-O-methyltransferase: significance in the development of 18F-PETT scanning agents", Biochemical and Biophysical Research Communications 130, 1123-1131.

Cumming, P., Boyes, B.E., Martin, W.R.W., Adam, M., Grierson, J., Ruth, T. and McGeer, E.G. (1987a) "The metabolism of [18F]6-Fluoro-L-3,4-dihydroxyphenylalanine in the hooded rat", J. Neurochem 48, 601-608.

Cumming, P., Boyes, B. E., Martin, W. R. W., Adam, M., Ruth, T.J. and McGeer, E.G. (1987b) "Altered metabolism of [18F]-6-Fluorodopa in the hooded rat following inhibition of catechol-O-methyltransferase with U-0521", Biochemical Pharmacology 36, 2527-2531.

Cumming, P., Häusser, M., Martin, W. R. W., Grierson, J., Adam, M. J., Ruth, T.J. and McGeer, E. G. (1988) "Kinetics of in vitro decarboxylation and the in vivo metabolism of 2-18F- and 6-18F-Fluorodopa in the hooded rat", Biochemical Pharmacology 37, 247-250.

Doller, H. J. and Connor, J. D. (1980) "Changes in neostriatal dopamine concentrations in response to levodopa infusions", J. Neurochem. 34, 1264-1269.

Firnau, G., Garnett, E. S., Chirakal, R., Sood, S., Nahmias, C. and Schrobilgen, G. (1986) "[18F]Fluoro-L-dopa for the in vivo study of intracerebral dopamine", Appl. Radiat. Isot. 37, 669-675.

Firnau, G., Sood, S., Chirakal, R., Nahmias, C. and Garnett, E. S. (1987) "Cerebral metabolism of 6-[F-18]Fluoro-L-dopa in the primate", J. Neurochem 48, 1077 -1082.

Firnau, G., Sood, S., Chirakal, R., Nahmias, C., Garnett, S. E. (1988) "Metabolites of 6-[18F]Fluoro-L-dopa in human blood", J. Nucl Med 29, 363-369.

Garnett, E.S., Firnau, G., Nahmias, C., Sood, S. and Belbeck, L. (1980) "Blood-brain barrier transport and cerebral utilization of dopa in living monkeys", Am. J. Physiol. 238, R318-R327.

Hefti, F., Melamed, E. and Wurtman, R. J. (1980) "The decarboxylation of DOPA in the parkinsonian brain: in vivo studies on an animal model", J. Neural Transmission 16,95-101.

Horne, M..K, Cheng, C.H. and Wooten, G.F. (1984) "The cerebral metabolism of L-dihydroxyphenylalanine. An autoradiographic and biochemical study", Pharmacology 28, 12-26.

Knudsen, G. M., Pettigrew, K. D., Patlak, C. S., Hertz, M. M. and Paulson, O. B. (1990) "Asymmetrical transport of amino acids across the blood-brain barrier in humans", J. Cerebral Blood Flow and Metabol. 10, 698-706.

Leenders, K. L., Palmer, A. J., Quinn, N., Clark, J. C., Firnau, G., Garnett, E. S., Nahmias, C., Jones, T. and Marsden, C. D. (1986a) "Brain dopamine metabolism in patients with Parkinson's disease measured with positron emission tomography", J. Neurol Neurosurg Psychiat 49, 853-856.

Leenders, K. L., Poewe, W. H., Palmer, A. J., Brenton, D. P. and Frackowiak, R. S. J. (1986b) "Inhibition of L-[^{18}F]fluorodopa uptake into human brain by amino acids demonstrated by positron emission tomography", Ann Neurol 20, 258-262.

Leenders, K. L., Salmon, E. P., Turton, D., Tyrrell, P., Perani, D., Brooks, D. J., Sagar, H., Jones, T., Marsden, C. D. and Frackowiak, R. S. J. (1990) "The nigro-striatal dopaminergic system assessed in vivo by positron emission tomography in healthy volunteer subjects and patients with Parkinson's disease", Archives of Neurology 47,1290-1298

Lloyd, K. G., Hockmann, C. H., Davidson, L., Farley, I.J. and Hornykiewicz, O. (1980) "Kinetics of L-DOPA metabolism in the caudate nucleus of cats with ventrotegmental lesions", J. of Neural Transmission suppl 16, 33- 44.

Melega, W. P., Hoffman, J. M., Luxen, A., Nissenson, C. H. K., Phelps, M. E. and Barrio, J. R. (1990a) "The effects of carbidopa on the metabolism of 6-[18F]fluoro-L-dopa in rats, monkeys and humans", Life Sciences 47, 149-157.

Melega, W. P., Luxen, A., Perlmutter, M. M., Nissenson, C. H. K., Phelps, M. E. and Barrio, J. R. (1990b) "Comparative in vivo metabolism of 6-[18F]fluoro-L-dopa and [3H]L-dopa in rats", Biochemical Pharmacology 39, 1853-1860.

Patlak, C. S., Blasberg, R. G. and Fenstermacher, J. D. (1983) "Graphical evaluation of Blood-to-brain transfer constants from multiple-time uptake data", J. Cereb Blood Flow Metabol 3, 1-7.

Patlak, C. S. and Blasberg, R. G. (1985) "Graphical evaluation of blood-to-brain transfer constants from multiple-time uptake data. Generalizations", J. Cereb Blood Flow Metabol 5, 584-590.

Reith, J., Dyve, S., Kuwabara, H., Guttman, M., Diksic, M. and Gjedde, A. (1990) "Blood-brain transfer and metabolism of 6-[18F]fluoro-L-dopa in rat", J. Cerebral Blood Flow and Metabolism 10, 707-719.

Sawle, G., Colebatch, J.G., Shah, A., Brooks, D.J., Marsden, C.D., and Frackowiak, R.S.J. (1990) "Striatal function in normal aging: implication for Parkinson's disease", Annals of Neurology 28, 799- 804.

Wade, L. A. and Katzman, R. (1975) "3-O-methyldopa uptake and inhibition of L-dopa at the blood-brain barrier", Life Sciences 17, 131-136.

DOPAMINE REUPTAKE SITES: THE ISSUES

E. SALMON

ABSTRACT. Although the mechanism of monoamine reuptake is a well established important phenomenon, the singleness or coexistence of monoamine transporter and reuptake inhibitor binding site is still discussed, and little is known about the physiological or drug regulation of that structure. Ligands for visualizing the monoaminergic reuptake sites are available for positron emission tomography. The reuptake sites can be taken, both in vitro and in vivo, as markers of the monoaminergic neuron terminal density. But positron emission tomography should also allow to assess the in vivo regulation of the binding sites and the kinetics of ligands binding which can be relevant to clinical symptoms.

1. Introduction

Positron emission tomography allows to perform in vivo studies of the neurotransmission pathways. While there are numerous ligands for many different post-synaptic receptors, the markers for the pre-synaptic side are very few. Presynaptic reuptake systems play an important physiological and pathological role, both in neurological and psychiatric disorders, for they transport, for example, monoamines and structurally related compounds into the nerve terminals. In vitro studies did not allow to fully characterize the structure and the function of the dopamine reuptake sites, but radiolabelled ligands are available to visualize them with positron emission tomography. The basic knowledge of the reuptake sites is first reviewed in this article, introducing, in a second part, the issues of PET studies.

2. The monoaminergic reuptake sites

Axelrod (1971) first demonstrated the mechanism of presynaptic reuptake for noradrenaline. The author observed in the rat an accumulation of tritiated noradrenaline in tissues with a high sympathetic innervation. This accumulation disappeared after section of the sympathetic nerves, while the physiological effects of the administration of noradrenaline were increased. It was suggested that a presynaptic reuptake system was responsible for a physiological inactivation of the neurotransmitter.

J. C. Baron et al. (eds.), Brain Dopaminergic Systems: Imaging with Positron Tomography, 111–119.

2.1. LABELING THE REUPTAKE SITES

Axelrod (1971) also showed that tricyclic antidepressants are able to inhibit the reuptake of monoamines. The radiolabelled drugs bind in vitro to the presynaptic neuron terminals. Comparative characteristics of some dopamine reuptake inhibitors are given in Table 1. Also more potent and more selective for labeling the dopamine reuptake site, [3H]GBR 12935 and the other derivatives of aryl-dialkylpiperazines also bind in all brain areas to piperazine acceptor sites (Andersen, 1987; de Keyser et al, 1989), which appear to be a form of cytochrome P450 enzyme (Niznik et al, 1990). A close parallelism is observed between the subcellular localization profile for [3H]dopamine reuptake and for [3H]GBR 12935 specific binding to dopamine reuptake sites in rat striatum (Maloteaux et al, 1988). When comparing different drugs (tricyclic antidepressants and others), their potency to bind to the reuptake sites is parallel to their capacity for inhibiting the neurotransmitter reuptake (Javitch et al, 1984). Surprisingly enough, the native neurotransmitter is a relatively poor competitor for the presynaptic binding. This could suggest the existence of a monoaminergic reuptake complex, where the monoamine transporter per se is coupled to a binding site accessible to drugs (Kennedy and Hanbauer, 1983; Dubocovich and Zahniser, 1985; Langer et al, 1987). However, the kinetics for monoamine binding and reuptake are likely to differ from that for reuptake inhibitors binding. A single site model remains possible, where the differences between reuptake inhibitors could be related to additional bonds outside the substrate recognition site (Andersen, 1989; Marcusson and Ross, 1990). Using photoaffinity labeling with 1-(2-[bis-(4-fluorophenyl)-methoxylethyl)-4-(2-[4-azido-3-[125I]iodophenyl]ethyl)piperazine ([125I]FAPP), Sallee et al (1989) identified the ligand binding subunit of the dopamine reuptake complex as an apparent 62kDA complex type glycoprotein. As stated by the authors, "molecular biological techniques will lead to determine the number of unique molecules" in the reuptake complexes, and "final assessment will await the purification of dopamine uptake site and its functional reconstitution and/or the isolation of cDNA clone encoding its synthesis".

2.2. PHYSIOLOGICAL REGULATION OF REUPTAKE SITES

Little is known about the physiological regulation of the reuptake sites. They are located both on axons and dendrites: Marcusson and Eriksson (1988) observed on the human brain in vitro that the highest binding of [3 H]GBR 12935 is to dopamine reuptake sites in the putamen and caudate nucleus, but with a relatively high binding in the substantia nigra as well. The fact that the proportion of [3 H]mazindol dopaminergic binding sites versus dopamine content is relatively higher in the substantia nigra pars compacta than in the caudate-putamen may reflect an ongoing synthesis of reuptake complexes in the endoplasmic reticulum of the cell body (Javitch et al , 1985). Circadian changes were described for 5-hydroxytryptamine (5HT) uptake in the rat hypothalamus and suprachiasmatic nucleus regions (Meyer and Quay, 1976), and for [3H]imipramine binding in the rat suprachiasmatic nucleus (Wirz-Justice et al, 1983). Langer et al (1987) postulated that the [3 H]imipramine binding site is a physiological relevant site, associated with and modulating the 5HT uptake site, and that it could be modulated by an endogenous ligand. However, that hypothesis has been questioned (Marcusson and Ross, 1990).

2.3. DRUG REGULATION OF REUPTAKE SITES

Drug regulation of the reuptake sites remains poorly understood. Palacios et al (1987) considered the general decrease in the density of the [3 H]imipramine binding sites they observed in the brain of patients chronically treated with this antidepressant as an example of brain receptor plasticity, and Plenge et al (1990) gave the same explanation to the decrease in [3 H]imipramine and [3H]paroxetine (another 5HT reuptake inhibitor) binding they observed in post mortem brain samples of a patient whith a long term lithium treatment. Some treatments of depression (antidepressants, rapid eye movement sleep deprivation, electroconvulsive therapy) were previously shown to down regulate [3 H]imipramine binding in the rat brain (Kinnier et al, 1980; Mogilnicka et al, 1980; Raisman et al, 1980), but since haloperidol induces down regulation of [3H]imipramine binding as well (Hrdina, 1984), and since the specific binding of the drug to 5HT reuptake sites was not determined, the functional significance of this down regulation is uncertain. Moreover, Langer et al (1987) suggested that there is a state dependent decrease of the brain and platelets [3H]imipramine binding sites in untreated depressed patients. Graham et al (1987) could not find any modification of the specific binding of [3 H]paroxetine to membrane fraction of cerebral cortex or hippocampus in rats after either acute or chronic treatment with specific inhibitors of the reuptake of 5HT or monoamine oxidase inhibitors. However, Scheffel and Hartig (1988) reported an upregulation of 5HT reuptake sites (labeled with [3 H]paroxetine) after eight days of MDMA (3,4-methylenedioxy-meth-amphetamine) treatment in mice, whereas a higher dose regimen has a toxic effect on 5HT axons, and reduces the density of [3 H]paroxetine-labeled 5HT reuptake complexes in rats (Battaglia et al, 1987; Commins et al, 1987).

Lee et al (1983) observed in the rat a regulation of the norepinephrine (NE) reuptake site by the neurotransmitter. Depletion of norepinephrine with reserpine reduced the number of reuptake sites (labelled with [3 H]desipramine, an inhibitor of NE reuptake), whereas increasing the concentration of NE by treatment with monoamine oxidase inhibitors raised this number. The authors proposed that "these dynamic alterations in norepinephrine uptake recognition sites may regulate synaptic function homeostatically".

Concerning the dopamine reuptake sites, [3H]GBR 12935 binding in rat is unaltered after chronic treatment with dopamine agonist and antagonist (Allard et al, 1990), while the administration of the monoamine oxidase inhibitor L-deprenyl in mice induces an upregulation of [3H]mazindol binding (Wiener et al, 1989).

2.4. MONOAMINERGIC REUPTAKE SITES AND DENSITY OF NERVE TERMINALS

The possible regulation of reuptake sites by neurotransmitters or by drugs is thus a complex problem that must be taken into account for PET studies. In most cases, however, monoamine uptake complexes are taken as a measure of the monoaminergic nerve terminals density (Sachs et al, 1975). Wagner et al (1980) demonstrated in the rat a loss of dopamine reuptake sites in the striatum after amphetamine administration, latter related to destruction of DA terminals (Ricaurte et al, 1984). There is a reduction of [3 H]mazindol binding sites in striatal membranes following destruction of dopaminergic neurons by 6-hydroxydopamine (Javitch et al, 1984), and a reduction of the specific binding of [3 H]threo-(±)-methylphenidate (inhibitor of dopamine reuptake) to rat striatum membranes following surgical lesions of the medial forebrain bundle (Janowsky et al, 1985).

In man, Zelnik et al (1986) found a significant decrease of [3 H]GBR-12935 binding sites in samples of caudate nucleus with age, which was explained as a progressive loss of dopaminergic neurons. There is a decrease in [3H]cocaine (Pimoule et al, 1983) and [3 H]GBR 12935 binding (Janowsky et al, 1987) to the caudate dopamine reuptake sites in Parkinson's disease, and Maloteaux et al (1988) also showed an important decrease of [3 H]GBR 12935 binding in the caudate nucleus and putamen of subjects with Parkinson's disease and progressive supranuclear palsy. Niznik et al (1991) reported a decrease of [125I]FAPP photoincorporation into the ligand functional neurons, some of those lacking tyrosine hydroxylase (Hirsch et al, 1988). From a clinical point of view, an inverse correlation has been found between [11 C]nomifensine specific uptake in the striatum and the severity of the akineto-rigid syndrome (Leenders et al, 1990).

3.2. [11C]COCAINE

[N-11C-methyl]-(-)-cocaine brain binding is the highest in the corpus striatum and the lowest in the cerebellum (Fowler et al, 1989). A possible drawback of using cocaine as a ligand is that it binds to dopaminergic, noradrenergic and serotoninergic reuptake complexes. Reith et al (1985, 1986) suggested that cortical cocaine sites and sodium-independent striatal cocaine binding sites are associated with 5HT transporters, on the basis of their sensitivity to the serotoninergic toxin 5,7-dihydroxytryptamine, while only sodium-sensitive cocaine sites are decreased in the striatum after lesions with the dopaminergic toxin 6-hydroxydopamine (Kennedy and Hanbauer, 1983). In PET experiments, pretreatment with nomifensine reduces the striatal uptake down to the cerebellar values, indicating that [11 C]cocaine binds to the dopaminergic reuptake sites, while pretreatment of two volunteers with desipramine did not change the relative distribution of [11 C]cocaine between striatum and cerebellum (Fowler et al, 1989).
There is an interesting parallelism between the [11 C]cocaine uptake time course in the striatum and the subjective feeling following cocaine intravenous administration, suggesting that the regional cocaine binding to the corpus striatum may be related to the neurochemical events which produce euphoria. This should allow to investigate the mechanisms responsible for cocaine's reinforcing properties, which in part involve the brain's dopamine systems (Galloway, 1988).
Beside the cocaine receptors on striatal dopamine reuptake complexes (Ritz et al, 1987) however, the medial prefrontal cortex (Goeders and Smith, 1983), the nucleus accumbens (Missale et al, 1985) are also said to support initiation of cocaine self-administration in rodents. In this connection, a consideration that deserves an explanation is that in vitro cocaine sodium-sensitive binding is specific for striatal sites, and cannot be detected in the nucleus accumbens for example (Missale et al, 1985), whereas [3H]GBR 12935 exhibits a specific high affinity binding in both striatum and nucleus accumbens (Berger et al, 1990).
Finally, a graphical analysis of [11C]cocaine plasma and tissue curves provides an estimation of the binding potential of the drug (Logan et al, 1990).

4. Conclusions

The study of the monoaminergic reuptake mechanism per se is not presently accessible to positron emission tomography, but drugs binding to the reuptake sites are available. To date, most of the in vitro and in vivo studies took the reuptake-binding sites as markers of monoaminergic terminals density, and the ligands allow to assess the loss of nigro-striatal dopaminergic neurons, both in experimental animals and in humans (Leenders et al, 1988; Salmon et al, 1990).

Although the fundamental relationship between the different tracers, their binding site(s) and the reuptake mechanism has still to be clarified, in vivo pharmacological challenges in primates and humans allow to characterize the binding properties. There are very few informations concerning a possible endogenous regulation of the reuptake sites and preliminary data show a good reproducibility of PET measurements. Short term modifications of reuptake complexes density after physiological or pharmacological challenge could be difficult to differentiate from modifications of drug binding possibilities, but delayed reuptake complexes regulation could be assessed in vivo with PET.

Finally, the kinetic of tracer uptake may be relevant to clinical symptoms (Fowler et al, 1989).

5. References

Allard, P., Eriksson, K., Ross, S.B., Marcusson, J.O. (1990) 'Unaltered [3H]GBR-1295 binding after chronic treatment with dopamine active drugs', Psychopharmacology, 102, 291-294.

Andersen, P.H., Jansen, J.A., Nielsen, E.B. (1987) '[3H]GBR 12935 binding in vivo in mouse brain: labelling of a piperazine acceptor site', Eur J Pharmacol, 144, 1-6.

Andersen, P.H. (1989) 'The dopamine uptake inhibitor GBR 12909: selectivity and molecular mechanism of action', Eur J Pharmacol, 166, 493-504.

Aquilonius, S.-M., Bergström, K., Eckernäs, S.A., Hartvig, P., Leenders, K.L., Lundquist, H., Antoni, G., Gee, A., Rimland, A., Uhlin, J., Langström, B. (1987) 'In vivo evaluation of striatal dopamine reuptake sites using 11C-nomifensine and positron emission tomography', Acta Neurol Scand, 76, 283-287.

Axelrod, J. (1971) 'Noradrenaline: fate and control of its biosynthesis', Science, 173, 598-606.

Battagllia, G., Yeh, S.I., O'Hearn, E., Molliver, M.E., Kuhar, M.J., De Souza, E.B. (1987) '3,4-methylenedioxymethamphetamine and 3,4-methylenedioxyamphetamine destroy serotonin terminals in rat brain: quantification of neurodegeneration by measurement of [3H]paroxetine labeled serotonin uptake sites',. J Pharmacol exp Ther, 242, 911-916.

Berger, .P, Elsworth, J.D., Arroyo, J., Roth, R.H. (1990) 'Interaction of [3H]GBR 12935 and GBR 12909 with the dopamine uptake complex in nucleus accumbens', Eur J Pharmacol, 177, 91-94.

Commins, D.L., Vosmer, G., Virus, R.M., Woolverton, W.L., Schuster, C.R., Seiden, L.S. (1987) 'Biochemical and histological evidence that methylenedioxymethamphetamine (MDMA) is toxic to neurons in the rat brain', J Pharmacol Exp Ther, 241, 338-345.

Davis, G.C., Williams, A.C., Markey, S.P., Ebert, M.H., Caine, E.D., Reichert, C.M., Kopin, I.J. (1979) 'Chronic parkinsonism secondary to intravenous injection of meperidine analogues', Psychiat Research, 1, 249-254.

De Keyser, J., De Backer, J.P., Ebinger, G., Vauquelin, G. (1989) '[3H]GBR 12935 binding to dopamine uptake sites in the human brain', J Neurochem, 53, 1400-1404.

Dubocovich, M.L., Zahniser, N.R. (1985) 'Binding characteristics of the dopamine uptake inhibitor [3H]nomifensine to striatal membranes', Biochem Pharmacol, 34, 1137-1144.

Fowler, J.S., Volkow, N.D., Wolf, A.P., Dewey, S.L., Schlyer, D.J., MacGregor, R.R., Hitzemann, R., Logan, J., Bendriem, B., Gatley, J., Christman, D. (1989) 'Mapping cocaine binding sites in human and baboon brain in vivo', Synapse, 4, 371-377.

Galloway, M.P. (1988) 'Neurochemical interactions of cocaine with dopaminergic systems', TIPS, 91, 451-454.

German, D.C., Manaye, K., Smith, W.K., Woodward, D.J., Saper, C.B. (1989) 'Midbrain dopaminergic cell loss in Parkinson's disease: computer visualization', Ann Neurol, 26, 507-514.

Goeders, N.E., Smith, J..E (1983) 'Cortical dopaminergic involvement in cocaine reinforcement', Science, 221, 773-775.

Graham, D., Tahraoui, L., Langer, S.Z. (1987) 'Effect of chronic treatment with selective monoamine oxidase inhibitors and specific 5-HT uptake inhibitors on [3H]paroxetine binding to cerebral cortical memebranes of the rat', Neuropharmacology, 26, 1087-1092.

binding subunit of the dopamine reuptake complex in parkinsonian postmortem caudate and no detectable photoincorporation in patients putamen.

3. Dopaminergic reuptake sites studied with positron emission tomography

Among the various markers of dopamine reuptake sites, [11C]nomifensine and [11C]cocaïne have been used for positron emission tomographic studies. There are also preliminary studies with piperazine derivatives such as [18 F]GBR 13119, which is mainly distributed in the striatal area in monkey brain (Kilbourn, 1989), and [18F]GBR 12909 (Koeppe et al, 1990; Stone-Elander et al, 1990).

3.1. [11C]NOMIFENSINE

Nomifensine is a potent inhibitor of both noradrenaline and dopamine reuptake by presynaptic neuronal terminals (Dubocovitch and Zahniser, 1985). Following intravenous administration of [11C]nomifensine in the rhesus monkey, the highest radioactivity uptake occurs in the striatum and the lowest in the cerebellum (Aquilonius et al, 1987). The ratio of the radioactivity between those two structures is markedly reduced after pretreatment with nomifensine or mazindol, whereas desipramine induces no change. After a unilateral lesion of the dopaminergic nigro-striatal pathway in a rhesus monkey by slowly infusing 1-methyl-4-phenyl-1,2,3,6-tetrahydropyridine (MPTP) into the right internal carotid artery, the specific binding of [11C]nomifensine in the lesioned striatum studied with PET disappears to a large extend, up to 80-90% (Leenders et al, 1988). Those observations suggest that the striatal signal obtained after [11C]nomifensine administration corresponds to dopaminergic reuptake sites, and that binding to noradrenergic neuron terminals or to glia is of little importance.

The brain distribution of [11C]nomifensine in volunteers shows a striking contrast between the high ligand uptake in striatum and the absence of detectable specific binding in frontal areas (Salmon et al, 1990), and this is in agreement with in vitro studies of [3H]GBR12935 distribution in human brain (Marcusson and Eriksson, 1988; de Keyser et al, 1989). This difference in density of reuptake sites between the nigro-striatal and the meso-cortical dopaminergic systems could be an explanation for the predominant vulnerability of the nigral pars compacta to MPTP (Davis et al, 1979; Salmon and Brooks, 1991).

Regional cerebral [11C]nomifensine uptake can be described with a conventional two-compartment model, providing a partition coefficient for the tracer between specific and nonspecific compartments (Salmon et al, 1990). The partition coefficient represents the binding potential of [11C]nomifensine to dopaminergic or noradrenergic uptake sites. In the putamen of patients suffering from Parkinson's disease or multiple system atrophy, the binding potential is similarly decrease to 40% of the control value. An influence of chronic levodopa therapy is very unlikely, since patients with multiple system atrophy received no dopaminergic drugs, so that [11C]nomifensine binding was taken as a marker of dopaminergic neuron terminal density (Leenders et al, 1990). The 40% value is very similar to that obtained in vitro with [3 H]GBR-12935 (Maloteaux et al, 1988) or in vivo with PET and [18F]fluorodopa (Leenders et al, 1990). It is compatible to the loss of substantia nigra dopaminergic neurons observed in anatomopathological studies (German et al, 1989). But the value is in striking contrast to dopamine levels measured postmortem in parkinsonian striatum, falling under 20% of control values. A possible explanation is that some of the remaining dopaminergic neurons are indeed non

Hirsch, E., Graybiel, A.M., Agid, Y.A. (1988) 'Melanized dopaminergic neurons are differentially susceptible to degeneration in Parkinson's disease',. Nature, 334, 345-348.
Hrdina, P..D (1984) '3H-imipramine binding sites in brain down regulated by chronic nortriptyline and haloperidol but not mianserin treatment', Psychiat Res, 11, 271-278.
Janowski, A., Schweri, M.M., Berger, P., Long, R., Skolnick, P., Paul, S.M. (1985) 'The effect of surgical and chemical lesions on striatal [3H]threo-(±)-methylphenidate binding, correlation with [3H]dopamine uptake', Eur J Pharmacol, 108, 187-191.
Janowski, A.A., Vocci, F., Berger, P., Angel, I., Zelnik, N., Kleinman, J.E., Skolnick, P., Paul, S.M. (1987) '[3H]GBR-12935 binding to the dopamine transporter is decreased in the caudate nucleus in Parkinson's disease', J Neurochem, 49, 617-621.
Javitch, J.A., Blaustein, R.O., Snyder, S.H. (1984) '[3H]mazindol binding associated with neuronal dopamine and norepinephrine uptake sites', Mol Pharmacol, 26, 35-44.
Javitch, J.A., Strittmatter, S.M., Snyde, S.H. (1985) 'Differential visualization of dopamine and norepinephrine uptake sites in rat brain using [3H]mazindol autoradiography', J Neurosci, 5, 1513-1521.
Kennedy, L.T., Hanbauer, I. (1983) 'Sodium sensitive cocaine binding to rat striatal membranes, possible relationship to dopamine uptake sites', J Neurochem, 41, 172-178.
Kilbourn, M.R., Carey, J.E., Koeppe, R.A., Haka, M.S., Hutchins, G.D., Sherman, P.S., Kuhl, D.E. (1989) 'Biodistribution, dosimetry, metabolism and monkey PET studies of [18F]GBR 13119. Imaging the dopamine uptake system in vivo', Nucl Med Biol, 16, 569-576.
Kinnier, W.J., Chuang, D.M., Costra, E. (1980) 'Down regulation of dehydroalprenolol and imipramine binding sites in brain of rats repeatedly treated with imipramine', Eur J Pharmacol, 67, 289- 291.
Koeppe, R.A., Kilbourn, M.R., Frey, K.A., Penney, J.B., Haka, M.S., Kuhl, D.E. (1990) 'Imaging and kinetic modeling of [F-18]GBR 12909, a dopamine uptake inhibitor', J Nucl Med, 31, 720.
Langer, S.Z., Galzin, A.M., Poirier, M.F., Loo, H., Sechter, D., Zarifian, E. (1987) 'Association of [3H]imipramine and [3H]paroxetine binding with the 5HT transporter in brain and platelets, relevance to depression', J Receptor Res, 7, 499-521.
Lee, C..M, Javitch, J..A, Snyder, S..H (1983) 'Recognition sites for norepinephrine uptake, regulation by neurotransmitter', Science, 220, 626-629.
Leenders,.. KL, Aquilonius, S.M., Bergström, K., Bjurling, P., Crossman, A..R, Eckernäs, S.A., Gee, A., Hartvig, P., Lundquist, H., Langström, B., Rimland, A., Tedroff, J. (1988) 'Unilateral MPTP lesion in a rhesus monkey, effect on the striatal dopaminergic system measured in vivo with PET using various novel tracers', Brain Res, 445, 61-67.
Leenders, K.L., Salmon, E., Tyrrel, P., Perani, D., Brooks, D.J., Sagar, H.J., Jones, T., Marsden, C.D., Frackowiak, R.S.J. (1991) 'The nigrostriatal dopaminergic system assessed in vivo by positron emission tomography in healthy volunteer subjects and patients with Parkinson's disease', Arch Neurol, 47, 1290-1298.
Logan, J., Fowler, J.S., Volkow, N.D., Wolf, A.P., Dewey; S..L, Schlyer, D.J., MacGregor, R.R., Hitezmann, R., Bendriem, B., Gatley, S.J., Christman, D.R. (1990) 'Graphical analysis of reversible radioligand binding from time-activity measurements applied to [N-11C-methyl]-(-)-cocaine PET studies in human subjects', J Cereb Blood Flow Metab, 10, 740-747.
Maloteaux, J.M., Vanisberg, M.A., Laterre, C., Javoy-Agid, F., Agid, Y., Laduron, P.M. (1988) '[3H]GBR 12935 binding to dopamine uptake sites, subcellular localization and reduction in Parkinson's disease and progressive supranuclear palsy', Eur J Pharmacol, 156, 331-340.
Marcusson,. J, Eriksson, K. (1988) '[3H]GBR-12935 binding to dopamine uptake sites in the human brain', Brain Res, 457, 122-129.

Marcusson, J..O, Ross, S..B (1990) 'Binding of some antidepressants to the 5-hydroxydopamine transporter in brain and platelets', Psychopharmacology, 102, 145-155.
Meyer, D..C, Quay, W.B. (1976) 'Hypothalamic and suprachiasmatic uptake of serotonin in vitro, twenty-four hour changes in male and prooestrus female rats', Endocrinol, 98, 1160-1165.
Missale, C., Castelletti, 1., Govoni, S., Spano, P..F, Trabucchi, M., Hanbauer, I. (1985) 'Dopamine uptake is differentially regulated in rat striatum and nucleus accumbens', J Neurochem, 45, 51-56.
Mogilnicka, E., Arbilla, S., Depoortere, H., Langer, S..Z (1980) 'Rapid eye movement sleep deprivation decreases the density of 3H-dehydroalprenolol and 3H-imipramine binding sites in the rat cerebral cortex', Eur J Pharmacol, 65, 289-292.
Niznik, H.B., Tyndale, R.F., Sallee, F.R., Gonzalez, F.J., Hardwick, J.P., Inaba, T., Kalow, W. (1990) 'The dopamine transporter and cytochrome P450IID1 (debrisoquine 4-hydroxylase) in brain, resolution and identification of two distinct [3H]GBR-12935 binding proteins', Arch Biochem Biophys, 276, 424-432.
Niznik, H..B, Fogel, E..F, Fassos, F.F., Seeman, P. (1991) 'The dopamine transporter is absent in parkinsonian putamen and reduced in the caudate nucleus', J Neurochem, 56, 192-198.
Palacios, J.M., Cortes, R., Probst, A. (1987) 'Receptor plasticity in the human brain, some autoradiographic studies', J Receptor Res, 7, 581-597.
Pimoule, C., Schoemaker, H., Javoy-Agid, F., Scatton, B., Agid, Y., Langer, S.Z. (1983) 'Decrease in 3H-cocaine binding to the dopamine transporter in Parkinson's disease', Eur J Pharmacol, 95, 145-146.
Plenge, P., Mellerup, E.T., Laursen, H. (1990) 'Regional distribution of the serotonin transport complex in human brain, identified with 3H-paroxetin, 3H-citalopram and 3H-imipramine', Prog Neuro-Psychopharmacol, 14, 61-72.
Raisman, R., Briley, M., Langer, S.Z. (1980) 'Specific tricyclic antidepressant binding sites in rat brain characterised by high-affinity 3H-imipramine binding', Eur J Pharmacol, 61, 373-376.
Reith, M.E., Meisler, B.E., Sershen, H., Lajtha, A. (1985)' Sodium independent binding of [3H]cocaine in mouse striatum is serotonin related', Brain Res, 342, 145-148.
Reith, M.E., Sershen, H., Lajtha, A. (1986) 'Binding sites for [3H]cocaine in mouse striatum and cerebral cortex have different dissociation kinetics', J Neurochem, 46, 309-312.
Ricaurte, G.A., Guillery, R.W., Seiden, L..S, Schuster, C.R. (1984) 'Nerve terminal degeneration after a single dose od D-amphetamine in iprindole-treated rats, relation to selective long lasting dopamine depletion', Brain Res, 291, 378-382.
Ritz, M..C, Lamb, R.J., Goldberg, S.R., Kuhar, M.J. (1987) 'Cocaine receptors on dopamine transporters are related to self-administration of cocaine', Science, 237, 1219-1223.
Sachs, C., Jonsson, G. (1975) 'Effect of 6-hydroxydopamine on central noradrenaline neurons during ontogeny', Brain Res, 99, 277-291.
Sallee, F..R, Fogel, E.L., Schwartz, E., Choi, S.M., Curran, D.P., Niznik, H.B. (1989) 'Photoaffinity labeling of the mammalian dopamine transporter', FEBS Letters, 256, 219-224.
Scatton, B., Dubois, A., Dubocovich, M.L., Zahniser, N.R., Fagel, D. (1985) 'Quantitative autoradiography of 3H-nomifensine binding sites in rat brain', Life Sci, 36, 815-822.
Salmon, E., Brooks, D.J., Leenders, K.L., Turton, D.R., Hume, S.P., Cremer, J.E., Jones, T., Frackowiak, R.S.J. (1990) 'A two compartmental description and kinetic procedure for measuring regional cerebral [11C]nomifensine uptake using positron emission tomography', J Cereb Blood Flow Metab, 10, 307-316.
Salmon, E., Brooks, D.J. (1991) 'In vivo distribution of catecholamine reuptake sites in human brain gives clues to the physiopathology of MPTP-induced parkinsonism', J Neurol Neurosurg Psychiat, in press.

Scheffel, U., Hartig, P..R (1988) 'In vivo labelling of the serotonin uptake sites with [3H]paroxetine and effect of MDMA', Abstract Society for Neuroscience, 558.

Schoemaker, H., Pimoule, C., Arbilla, S., Scatton, B., Javoy-Agid, F., Langer, S.Z. (1985) 'Sodium dependant [3H]cocaine binding associated with dopamine uptake sites in the rat striatum and human putamen decrease after dopaminergic denervation and in Parkinson's disease', Naunyn-Schmiedeberg's Arch Pharmacol, 329, 227-235.

Stone-Elander, S.A., Roland, P.E., Hohlweg, R. (1990) 'Synthesis of [F-18]GBR 12909 for evaluation as a tracer for dopamine uptake inhibition', J Nucl Med, 31, 902.

Wagner, G.C., Ricaurte, G.A., Johanson, C.E., Schuster, C.R., Seiden, L.S. (1980) 'Amphetamine induces depletion of dopamine and loss of dopamine uptake sites in caudate , Neurology, 20, 547-550.

Wiener, H.L., Hashim, A., Lajtha, A., Sershen, H. (1989) 'Chronic L-deprenyl-induced up-regulation of the dopamine uptake carrier', Eur J Pharmacol, 163, 191-194.

Wirz-Justice, A., Krauchi, K., Morimasa, T., Willener, R., Feer, H. (1983)'Circadian rythm of [3H]imipramine binding in the rat suprachiasmatic nuclei', Eur J Pharmacol, 87, 331-333.

Zelnik, N., Angel, I., Paul, S.M., Kleinman, J.E. (1986) 'Decreased density of human striatal dopamine uptake sites with age', Eur J Pharmacol, 126, 175-176.

Movement Disorders: the clinical issues

David J. Brooks

Introduction

Preceeding chapters in this symposium have dealt with the various approaches to modelling striatal uptake of PET tracers of the dopaminergic system. The tracers ^{18}F-6-fluorodopa (FD) and ^{11}C-nomifensine (NMF) are useful for assessing the integrity of the presynaptic nigro-striatal dopaminergic system. Striatal FD uptake reflects striatal aromatic aminoacid decarboxylase (AADC) activity and dopamine storage capacity, while striatal NMF binding reflects dopamine reuptake site density. Integrity of striatal post-synaptic dopamine D_1 receptors can be studied with the tracers ^{11}C-SCH 23390 and ^{11}C-SCH 39166. Uptake of ^{11}C-raclopride (RAC), ^{76}Br-bromospiperone (BSP), ^{11}C-methylspiperone (MSP), ^{18}F-fluoro- spiperone, and ^{18}F-fluoroethylspiperone, all reflect D_2 site density.

PET provides a means not only of examining the patterns of alteration in dopaminergic function associated with movement disorders and the dementias, but also a potential means of detecting subclinical disruption of the dopaminergic system in at-risk subjects. In this chapter it is intended to consider the following questions: (1) Are PET studies on the dopaminergic system able to show selective patterns of disruption in different degenerative disorders leading to Parkinsonism (Parkinson's disease (PD), multiple system atrophy (MSA), progressive supranuclear palsy (PSP), corticobasal degeneration (CBD) ? (2) Can the development of fluctuating responses to L-dopa in PD, and the poor responses of MSA and PSP to dopamine agonists, be explained in terms of alterations in striatal dopamine receptor levels ? (3) Are conditions associated with involuntary movements (chorea, dystonia, dyskinesia, postural and rest tremor) associated with disruption of the dopaminergic system ? (4) Can PET detect subclinical abnormalities in nigrostriatal function in at-risk subjects for Parkinson's disease (the elderly, twins and relatives of affected PD patients, subjects exposed to nigral toxins, patients who develop severe rigidity taking convential doses of dopamine receptor blocking agents) ?

J. C. Baron et al. (eds.), Brain Dopaminergic Systems: Imaging with Positron Tomography, 121–134.

(1) The Parkinsonian syndromes

(a) Parkinson's disease

Parkinson's disease is characterised by Lewy body degeneration of the substantia nigra compacta. The ventrolateral nigral projections to the putamen are targeted, with more moderate degeneration of caudate dopaminergic nerve terminals. It has been estimated that by the onset of clinical symptoms putamen dopamine levels have fallen to less than 20% of normal. The first reports on striatal ^{18}F-Dopa uptake in PD were those of Garnett et al [1], and Nahmias et al [2]. Their subjects had hemiparkinsonism, and were early into the disease. PET showed preserved caudate, but bilaterally reduced putamen, ^{18}F uptake, activity being most depressed in the putamen contralateral to the affected limbs. These studies, therefore, confirmed that the pattern of disruption of the dopaminergic system predicted from pathological studies could be detected in-vivo in PD with PET. They were also the first demonstration that subclinical involvement of dopaminergic projections to the putamen contralateral to clinically unaffected limbs in PD could be detected.

Other groups have subsequently confirmed these observations [3-5], and demonstrated a significant correlation between depression in striatal ^{18}F-Dopa uptake of PD patients and their degree of locomotor disability [3,4]. Mean putamen ^{18}F-Dopa uptake in PD is reduced to 40% of normal. A 60-80% loss of nigra compacta cells and a 80-90% loss of putamen dopamine levels is found at post-mortem in PD [6]. It is likely, therefore, that striatal ^{18}F-Dopa uptake reflects functional integrity of nigro-striatal fibres rather than levels of endogenous striatal dopamine which are specifically determined by tyrosine hydroxylase activity.

As with ^{18}F-Dopa, mean specific putamen uptake of the active (+) enantiomer of ^{11}C-nomifensine, a dopamine re-uptake antagonist, is reduced to 40% of normal levels in PD, while caudate tracer uptake is relatively preserved [7]. Specific ^{11}C-NMF uptake by the putamen in individual PD patients correlates with both ^{18}F-Dopa uptake, and also with their locomotor function, confirming that both these tracers reflect functional integrity of nigro-striatal dopaminergic terminals [8].

^{11}C-raclopride is a highly selective, reversible dopamine D_2 receptor antagonist. Equilibrium striatal: cerebellum RAC uptake ratios reflect striatal D_2 site density. Rinne et al [9] measured striatal: cerebellum RAC uptake ratios in 7 untreated hemiparkinsonian patients (later shown to be L-Dopa responsive). They found a relative 10% mean increase in RAC uptake in the striatum contralateral to the affected limbs. We have confirmed this finding in a further 4 untreated hemiparkinsonian patients [10]. These subjects had serial ^{18}F-Dopa and RAC scans. ^{18}F-Dopa uptake was depressed, and RAC binding increased, in the putamen contralateral to the affected limbs, an inverse correlation between the binding of the two tracers being found.

While a 10-15% relative upregulation of D_2 sites appears appears to occur in the putamen contralateral to the affected limbs in untreated PD, we have found that absolute putamen: cerebellar RAC uptake ratios still fall within the normal range - see table 1. Leenders et al [11] also found normal levels of striatal ^{11}C-methylspiperone (MSP) binding binding in untreated PD. Post-mortem studies on untreated PD cases have reported both normal and raised levels of striatal D_2

receptors [12,13]. Nigral lesions in animals lead to 50% rises in striatal D_2 receptor densities over two weeks [14,15], but by one year these normalise again. Our untreated PD patients whose striatal:cerebellum ^{11}C-raclopride binding ratios lay within the normal range had a mean clinical disease duration of 2.6 years. It is conceivable that any initial upregulation of striatal D_2 sites that occurs in PD as a response to nigral degeneration later tends to reverse as adaptive mechanisms come into play.

(b) Multiple system atrophy

Multiple system atrophy (MSA), occasionally known as Shy-Drager syndrome, includes striatonigral degeneration (SND), olivopontocerebellar atrophy (OPCA), and progressive autonomic failure (PAF), in its spectrum. About 10% of cases initially diagnosed as Parkinson's disease have SND at autopsy [16]. The pathology of MSA is distinct from PD, and consists of neuronal loss from the basal ganglia, brain-stem and cerebellar nuclei, and intermediolateral columns of the cord, without neuronal inclusion body formation. As with PD, the ventrolateral nigra is targeted but nigral involvement can be diffuse (33). In its early stages MSA may be clinically difficult to distinguish from PD, as it can present as an akinetic-rigid syndrome which is initially L-Dopa responsive. Later the response to L-Dopa diminishes and cerebellar ataxia and severe autonomic failure become evident.

As with PD, akinetic-rigid MSA patients show a mean reduction of putamen ^{18}F-Dopa and ^{11}C-nomifensine uptake to 40% of normal levels, and individual levels of putamen ^{18}F-Dopa uptake correlate with locomotor function [4,17]. Caudate ^{18}F-Dopa and NMF uptake are significantly more depressed in MSA than PD [7,17], confirming a greater involvement of dorsomedial nigra in MSA. Table 1 shows mean striatal: cerebellum ^{11}C-raclopride uptake ratios in 8 patients with probable SND. It can be seen that their mean putamen RAC uptake was reduced to 87% of normal, in contrast to untreated PD patients who had normal putamen RAC uptake. It has been suggested that pure autonomic failure, olivopontocerebellar atrophy, and striatonigral degeneration are extremes of the spectrum comprising MSA. In our study 6 out of 7 patients with PAF had normal striatal FD uptake, while the seventh showed evidence of subclinical nigral involvement [17]. This finding would argue against PAF being in general a form fruste of MSA. At post-mortem OPCA patients may show evidence of sub-clinical SND, and SND patients of OPCA [16]. We have scanned three patients with sporadic OPCA (ataxia and autonomic failure, but no rigidity) [18]. All three had normal striatal FD uptake, suggesting that OPCA and SND may exist as separate variants of MSA on occassion.

(c) Progressive Supranuclear Palsy

This condition, (Steele-Richardson-Olszewski syndrome), is characterised pathologically by neuronal loss from the basal ganglia, superior colliculi, brainstem nuclei, and the periaqueductal grey matter with intraneuronal neurofibrillary tangle formation [19]. Unlike PD where ventrolateral nigra is selectively targeted, in PSP there is uniform involvement of nigro-striatal dopaminergic projections [20,21]. The condition is clinically manifested as an L-Dopa resistant akinetic-rigid syndrome, with axial rigidity, a supranuclear down-gaze palsy, bulbar dysfunction, and dementia of frontal type. Initially patients may present with a partially L-Dopa responsive akinetic-rigid syndrome in the absence of supranuclear gaze problems, making a distinction from PD difficult.

Table 1

Mean Equilibrium Striatal:Cerebellum ^{11}C-Raclopride Uptake Ratios in PD, SND, and PSP

		Caudate (mean±SD)	Putamen (mean±SD)
Controls	(8)	3.56±.35	3.60±.40
PD untreated	(6)	3.23±.33	3.42±.38
treated	(5)	**2.38±.41	**2.39±.22
SND	(8)	3.26±.47	*3.09±.29
PSP	(9)	*2.67±.69	3.22±.63

* $p < .02$ compared to normal } Student's t test
** $p < .005$ compared to normal

We have studied the integrity of the nigro-striatal dopaminergic projections in PSP with ^{18}F-Dopa [4]. In 10 patients mean putamen tracer uptake was reduced to 41%, and caudate to 48%, of normal levels. This finding contrasts with PD where caudate FD uptake was usually twice that of putamen, and confirms pathological observations that nigro-striatal fibres are globally affected in PSP. In our PSP patients, unlike PD and MSA, there was no correlation between levels of striatal ^{18}F-Dopa uptake and locomotor disability. This suggests that the rigidity and bradykinesia of PSP are determined by striatal and pallidal degeneration, rather than loss of dopaminergic neurons.

Integrity of striatal dopamine D_2 receptors in PSP has been studied with ^{76}Br-bromospiperone, ^{11}C-raclopride, and 18F-fluoroethylspiperone. Baron et al [22] found a mean 24% fall in equilibrium striatal:cerebellar BSP uptake ratio in seven PSP patients compared to age-matched normal controls. Six of these subjects, however, were on regular treatment with dopamine agonists and so treatment- induced D_2 downregulation could have influenced these authors findings. We have studied 9 PSP patients with ^{11}C-raclopride, 4 of whom were taking L-dopa or dopamine agonists. Table 1 shows that there was a 21% and 11% reduction in their caudate:cerebellum and putamen:cerebellum tracer RAC uptake, respectively, compared to normal controls. This pattern contrasts with that of SND where putamen RAC binding was more depressed than caudate. Only caudate FESP uptake has been reported in PSP. Wienhard et al [23] found a mean 17% fall in FESP caudate binding potential for their 2 PSP cases.

If it is assumed that cerebellar uptake of RAC reflects only non-specific tracer binding, and that PSP results in loss of D_2 site density without changing receptor affinity, it can be calculated that the 21% fall in the caudate:cerebellum RAC uptake ratio in PSP is equivalent to a 30% loss of caudate D_2 sites. This finding is in reasonable agreement with pathological studies where 30-48%, and 37-42%, losses of caudate and putamen D_2 binding sites have been reported [12,21].

(d) Corticobasal degeneration

This syndrome, also known as neuronal achromasia, corticodentatonigral degeneration, and corticobasalganglionic degeneration, presents with characteristic clinical features. Patients initially develope an akinetic-rigid, painful, dyspraxic or alien limb, with cortical sensory loss, and myoclonus. Supranuclear gaze palsy and bulbar dysfunction are also features of this condition, while intellect is characteristically spared [24]. Eventually the akinetic-rigid syndrome generalises, and response to L-Dopa is poor. The pathology consists of collections of swollen, achromatic, Pick cells, but without argyrophillic inclusion bodies, concentrated in posterior frontal, inferior parietal, and superior temporal cortex, in the cerebellar dentate nuclei, and in substantia nigra. Unlike PSP, the disease onset of CBD is strikingly asymmetric.

There has been only one PET study reported to date of dopaminergic function in patients with the clinical syndrome of CBD. Sawle et al [25] studied 6 patients and found that striatal ^{18}F-Dopa uptake was strikingly assymetrical, being most depressed contralateral to the more affected limbs. Unlike PD, but similar to PSP, caudate and putamen tracer uptake were equally severely depressed in CBD. Interestingly, these authors found that mesial frontal ^{18}F-Dopa uptake was also significantly depressed in CBD. This is not the case in PD, MSA, or PSP (Brooks DJ, unpublished observations).

To summarise, the different patterns of involvement of the dopaminergic system in the various degenerative disorders associated with Parkinsonism can be distinguished with PET. In PD there is sparing of nigro-caudate as compared to putamen dopaminergic projections, as evidenced by preserved levels of caudate FD and NMF uptake. In the multiple system degenerations PSP, and CBD, caudate and putamen projections are equally involved. MSA patients show mild to severe degrees of impaired caudate FD and NMF uptake. Striatal D_2 sites are preserved in untreated PD, but SND and PSP patients show reduced striatal binding of D_2 antagonists (RAC, BSP, FESP), putamen and caudate being targeted, respectively.

(2) L-dopa responsiveness and integrity of the dopaminergic system

It is currently unclear why patients with Parkinson's disease show an initial sustained response to L-dopa, but after some years develop fluctuating "on-off" and dyskinetic responses to this agent. Contributing factors are likely to include: (1) continued loss of striatal dopaminergic terminals resulting in a diminished dopamine storage and reuptake capacity. (2) variable absorption of L-dopa from the gut. (3) loss of striatal D_2 receptor responsiveness (either due to receptor loss or alterations in relative numbers of high and low affinity D_2 sub-populations).

PD patients with a fluctuating response to L-dopa have lower levels of striatal FD uptake than sustained responders [3]. Table 1 shows striatal:cerebellar RAC uptake ratios for a group of 5 PD patients with mean clinical disease duration 8 years all of whom had a fluctuating L-dopa response. It can be seen that there was a 30% fall in both caudate and putamen tracer binding. Leenders et al [11] noted a mean 20% decrease in striatum:cerebellum ^{11}C-MSP binding in five treated PD patients, and Wienhard et al [23] found a mean 18% decrease in caudate ^{18}F-fluoroethylspiperone (FESP) binding potential in 7 PD subjects. We are currently unable to tell whether the loss of D_2 binding sites in our fluctuating PD group reflects degeneration secondary to disease activity, or down-regulation due to prolonged treatment exposure.

At post-mortem treated PD patients have been reported to have normal or reduced levels of striatal D_2 receptors [12,26]. Only one pathological study analysed striatal D_2 density of treated PD patients as a function of their treatment response [27]. These workers found normal mean levels of striatal D_2 sites in sustained, and reduced levels in fluctuating responders, respectively, in agreement with our PET findings. There is evidence from animal work that both L-Dopa and dopamine agonists can down-regulate striatal D_2 sites. Fuxe et al [28] found a 25% fall in rat striatal dopamine receptors after two weeks of pergolide threatment, and Mishra [29] reported similar findings after three weeks of L-Dopa ingestion. In order to settle the issue of whether PD per se leads to loss of striatal D_2 sites serial PET studies following changes in D_2 density in untreated PD are required.

Table 1 shows that our SND and PSP patients showed a 13% and 11% fall in their mean putamen:cerebellum RAC uptake ratios, and caudate uptake was also reduced by 21% in PSP. Striatal:cerebellar RAC uptake ratios were reduced by 30% in fluctuating PD patients. It has been estimated that neuroleptic-induced rigidity only occurs after 80% striatal D_2 blockade [30]. The falls in striatal D_2 site density found in SND and PSP, therefore, are unlikely to be sufficient to explain the lack of L-dopa response of these patients, which is probably due to loss of other pallidal and brain-stem connections. On-off fluctuations in PD are also unlikely to be caused by a 30% fall in striatal D_2 density alone, but may well result from D_2 sites switching inappropriately from high to low affinity conformations. As D_2 antagonists bind with equal affinity to high and low affinity D_2 conformations PET is incapable at present of resolving this question.

(3) Involuntary Movements and the Dopaminergic System

(a) Tremor

It has been suggested that there may be a relationship between essential tremor and PD. 20% of relatives of PD patients have been said to have a postural tremor on examination, while 3-19% of patients with a sporadic postural tremor develop Parkinsonism [31-33]. There has also been debate over whether a benign tremulous form of PD exists where patients have a predominant rest tremor, but show little rigidity or akinesia for many years. We have studied striatal ^{18}F-Dopa uptake in 29 patients with isolated tremors, that is with no evidence of sustained rigidity or bradykinesia, cerebellar ataxia, or dystonic posturing. Ten patients had a predominant rest tremor, while 19 had

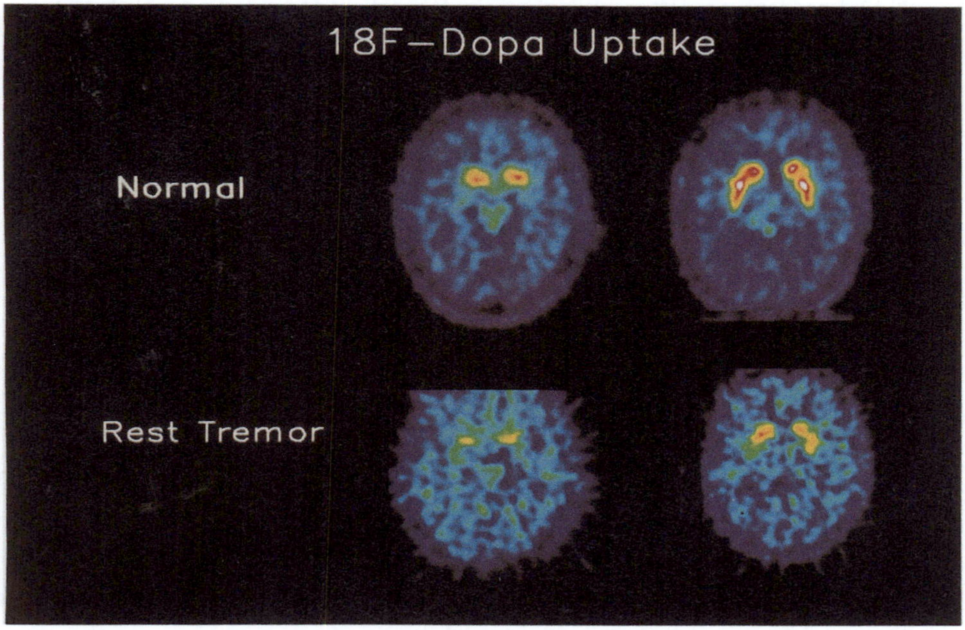

Fig. 1. PET images of striatal ^{18}F-dopa uptake 30-90 minutes after tracer administration in a normal subject and rest tremor patient. The patient shows severe loss of putamen and mild loss of head of caudate activity, similar to that in PD.

predominant postural tremor (8 familial and 11 sporadic).

The 8 subjects with a familial postural tremor all showed striatal ^{18}F-Dopa uptake within the normal range. All 10 subjects with a predominant rest tremor had subnormal putamen ^{18}F-Dopa uptake, nine subjects having influx constants falling within the PD range. As in PD, caudate FD uptake in the rest tremor patients was reletively spared. Fig 1 shows PET images of striatal FD uptake for one of these rest tremor patients. Nine of the 11 patients with sporadic postural tremor had normal striatal FD uptake, but two had subnormal levels of putamen activity, one falling into the PD range. This last subject has subsequently become akinetic. Table 2 details the mean striatal FD influx constants for these 3 groups of tremor patients, and a group of patients with sporadic PD. Our preliminary findings suggest that familial essential tremor is not associated with pathology of the nigro-striatal dopaminergic system. The presence of predominant rest tremor strongly correlates with reduced striatal ^{18}F-Dopa binding supporting the existence of a tremulous form of PD. The majority of patients with sporadic postural tremor have no evidence of nigral dysfunction.

(b) Chorea and Tardive Dyskinesia

The dopaminergic system has only been studied with PET in two choreiform syndromes: Huntington's disease (HD) and neuroacanthocytosis (NA). Leenders et al [34] scanned a single HD patient and noted normal striatal ^{18}F-Dopa uptake within the 1.7 cm resolution of their camera. Three groups have reported severely reduced striatal D_2 receptor density in HD, as evidenced

Table 2

Mean Striatal ^{18}F-Dopa influx constants (Ki min^{-1}) in Isolated Tremor

	Putamen (mean±SD)	Caudate (mean±SD)
Normals (30)	.0098±.0011	.0107±.0019
Familial (8)	.0085±.0009	.0099±.0011
Sporadic postural (11)	.0088±.0014	.0103±.0017
Sporadic rest (10)	*.0053±.0013	*.0083±.0016
PD (16)	*.0047±.0010	.0090±.0021

* $p< .05$ Bonferroni statistics

by low ^{11}C-methylspiperone (MSP) and FESP binding [23,35]. We have studied 6 patients with chorea due to Neuroacanthocytosis (NA) [36]. Caudate and anterior putamen ^{18}F-Dopa uptake were normal in the NA subjects, but posterior putamen tracer uptake was reduced to 40% of normal. Similar findings were seen in a subject with akinetic-rigid HD. Such a selective abnormality of posterior putamen ^{18}F-Dopa uptake in HD would be missed by a low resolution PET camera. Striatal D_2 site density, assessed with ^{11}C-raclopride, was reduced to 30% of normal levels in the NA patients. The similar pattern of disruption of the dopaminergic system found for HD and NA is not surprising as the nature of their striatal pathology is very similar despite their different aetiologies [37].

Although striatal D_2 receptor density is severely reduced in HD and NA, it is normal in tardive dyskinesia (TD) [38,39]. This finding argues against TD being due to striatal D_2 receptor supersensitivity, and primate models suggest that the condition is associated with 50% reductions in sub-thalamic nucleus levels of GABA.

(c) Dystonia

Non L-Dopa responsive idiopathic torsion dystonia (ITD) is thought to be a dominantly inherited condition with a 40% penetrance [40]. It has been linked to a gene deletion on chromosome 9 [41]. Dopa-responsive dystonia (DRD) is also familial, but has a different gene locus to ITD. Pathological studies have failed to identify any consistent abnormalities in ITD. Patients with aquired hemidystonia generally have lesions of the caudate, lentiform nucleus, or ventral thalamus [42].

A problem with PET studies reported to date on dystonia has been the heterogeneity of the patients examined. Familial, sporadic, and aquired dystonia has been considered en masse, and hemi- and focal dystonics have been frequently selected so that side-to-side comparisons of basal ganglia function can be made. As a consequence the relevance of PET findings to familial ITD remains unclear. Leenders et al [43] reported striatal ^{18}F-Dopa uptake in 4 patients with hemidystonia, and two patients with torticollis. 3 of his hemidystonic patients had dystonia-parkinsonism rather than ITD, and one of these 3 had a calcified lesion in the midbrain tegmentum. All 6 subjects showed abnormal striatal ^{18}F-Dopa uptake, and in the 4 hemidystonics this was most depressed in the striatum contralateral to the affected limbs. Three of the four hemidystonic patients had normal striatal MSP binding, while the fourth patient with a midbrain lesion showed striatal D_2 receptor upregulation secondary to the loss of nigro-striatal projections.

Playford et al [44] have examined striatal FD uptake in 12 ITD patients with a verifiable family history. Four of these 12 subjects showed subnormal levels of putamen FD uptake. There was no correlation between putamen FD influx constants and disease severity in these 12 subjects. The authors concluded that reduced putamen FD binding was probably an epiphenomenon with low penetrance in ITD, and unlikely to be the cause of the dystonic posturing.

Sawle et al [45] examined striatal ^{18}F-Dopa uptake in 6 subjects with clinically typical L-Dopa responsive dystonia (DRD). Four of the six subjects had striatal tracer uptake that was within the normal range, but the group as a whole showed a mean 25% fall in mean striatal ^{18}F-Dopa uptake. As all were taking regular L-dopa this may have led to down-regulation of striatal FD uptake. A seventh subject labelled as DRD, who required much larger and more frequent doses of L-dopa than the other six, had levels of putamen FD uptake in the PD range. Martin et al [46] studied striatal ^{18}F-Dopa uptake in four dystonic subjects. One had DRD and a normal level of striatal ^{18}F-Dopa uptake. The other three had ITD and two of these had impaired tracer binding.

Summary

Striatal FD uptake appears to be normal in familial essential tremor and most cases of sporadic postural tremor, but patients with isolated rest tremor show a PD pattern of impaired FD uptake, putamen being more affected than caudate. Chorea due to Huntington's disease or neuroacanthocytosis is associated with severe loss of striatal D_2 sites. To date the dopaminergic system in other causes of chorea has not been examined. Levels of striatal D_2 receptors are normal in tardive dyskinesia. Striatal FD uptake is inconsistently impaired in idiopathic torsion dystonia, and is probably an epiphenomenon with variable penetrance.

(4) Detection of sub-clinical nigral pathology

It has been estimated that patients do not develop symptoms of parkinsonism until they have lost over 50% of their nigra compacta cells, and 80% of their putamen dopamine [47]. Putamen FD uptake is reduced by at least 35% by the time of onset of tremor and rigidity [4] and so PET should provide a potential means of detecting sub-clinical pathology of the nigro-striatal dopaminergic system in at-risk subjects. Calne et al [48] first demonstrated this potential by PET scanning 4 asymptomatic subjects who had been exposed to MPTP and finding subnormal striatal FD uptake in 2 cases.

It has been suggested that Parkinson's disease may be caused by a sub-clinical toxic or infective insult in childhood, but only becomes clinically evident later when the nigral cell population falls below 50% of normal due to natural ageing [49]. In order to test this hypothesis two groups have studied striatal FD uptake in normal subjects over an age range of 20-80 years. The first group found a significant decline with age in 9 subjects [50], while the second larger study found no change with age in 30 subjects [51]. Recently the first group have reported that with additional numbers their age effect on striatal ^{18}F-Dopa uptake is less apparent. As post-mortem studies have shown evidence of a monocytic infiltration of the nigra in PD, indicative of an active inflammatory process, it is unlikely that ageing alone is responsible for the onset of parkinsonian symptoms [52].

The role of inheritance in PD is still unclear. Up to 41% of PD patients give a positive family history [53] and a member of one large kindred was recently shown to have Lewy-body nigral degeneration at post-mortem [54]. Initial twin studies, however, found a similar low concordance for PD among mono- and dizygotic twins and concluded that the disease was an acquired condition [55]. Recently, however, it has been suggested that these twin studies may have used diagnostic criteria for PD that were too narrow, and that with wider diagnostic criteria they do not exclude a genetic contribution to the etiology of PD. A problem with all epidemiological surveys into the incidence of PD is that sub-clinical cases will inevitably be scored as normal. PET should provide a potential means of detecting the presence of sub-clinical nigral pathology in at-risk relatives and twins of PD patients.

We have carried out ^{18}F-dopa PET on six monozygotic (MZ) and three dizygotic (DZ) PD co-twins to date [56]. Three of the 6 "unaffected" MZ, and two of the 3 "unaffected" DZ co-twins had one or both putamen FD influx constants reduced greater than 2 SD below the normal mean. Interestingly, two of the MZ twins with abnormal FD uptake who were said to be clinically unaffected had a postural tremor on examination. We have also studied a single PD kindred with four affected siblings who had putamen Ki values that were reduced to 38% (44yr M), 37% (40yr M), 31% (43yr F), and 33% (49yr M) of normal (data courtesy of Dr. GV Sawle). Putamen Ki values of an "unaffected" sibling (38yr M), and a daughter (19yr) of the 43 year old affected female were also significantly reduced to 48%, and 77%, of normal, respectively.

It has been suggested that dopamine receptor blocking agents (DRBA's) may act to unmask sub-clinical nigral pathology in patients who become rigid on conventional doses of these drugs. Two such patients were shown to have Lewy body nigral disease at post-mortem [57]. We have studied 7 cases with severe drug-induced parkinsonism (DIP) and no prior history suggestive of parkinsonism. Five of the 7 DIP patients had normal levels of striatal ^{18}F-Dopa uptake while two had putamen Ki values reduced more than 2 SD below the normal mean, one falling into the PD range. One year after PET 4 of the 5 subjects with normal striatal FD uptake have fully recovered on withdrawal of their DRBA's, while the 2 DIP patients with abnormal PET still require L-dopa. These findings would suggest that the majority of DIP cases do not have underlying nigral pathology.

Summary

PET measurements of striatal FD uptake are capable of revealing sub-clinical nigral pathology when this is present. Preliminary twin and kindred studies suggest that concordance for Parkinson's disease may be higher than was originally suspected. The current consensus is that there is no significant reduction in striatal FD uptake with age, which is against PD being caused by a childhood infective or toxic insult. Although dopamine receptor blocking agents may occassionally unmask latent PD, striatal FD uptake is generally normal in patients with drug-induced rigidity.

(5) Conclusions

In summary this section has shown that PET is capable of revealing the different patterns of disruption associated with different degenerative disorders causing parkinsonism, and with conditions causing involuntary movements. These functional changes can often be detected long before structural changes are evident on CT or MRI. PET can also detect sub-clinical involvement of the dopaminergic system in at-risk subjects for PD, and also potentially in at-risk subjects for HD, neuroacanthocytosis, and dystonia. Future developments may include the development of agonist as well as antagonist tracers so that high and low affinity receptor sub-populations can be quantitated in parkinsonian patients with a fluctuating or poor response to L-dopa.

References

[1] Garnett ES, Nahmias C, Firnau G (1984). Central dopaminergic pathways in hemiparkinsonism examined by positron emission tomography. Can. J. Neurol. Sci. 11, 174-179.

[2] Nahmias C, Garnett ES, Firnau G, Lang AE. (1985) Striatal dopamine distribution in Parkinsonian patients during life. J. Neurol. Sci. 11, 174-179.

[3] Leenders KL, Palmer AJ, Quinn N, et al. (1986) Brain dopamine metabolism in patients with Parkinson's Disease measured with positron emission tomography. J. Neurol. Neurosurg. Psychiat. 49, 853-860.

[4] Brooks DJ, Ibanez V, Sawle GV, et al. (1990) Differing patterns of Striatal ^{18}F-Dopa uptake in Parkinson's Disease, Multiple System Atrophy, and Progressive Supranuclear Palsy. Ann. Neurol. 28, 547-555.

[5] Martin WRW, Stoessl AJ, Adam MJ, et al. (1986) Positron Emission Tomography in Parkinson's Disease: Glucose and Dopa metabolism. Adv. Neurol. 45, 95-98

[6] German DC, Manaye K, Smith WK, Woodward DJ, Saper CB. (1989) Midbrain Dopaminergic Cell Loss in Parkinson's Disease: Computer Visualisation. Ann.Neurol. 26, 507-514.

[7] Salmon EP, Brooks DJ, Leenders KL, et al. (1990) A Two-Compartment Description and Kinetic Proceedure for measuring Regional Cerebral [^{11}C]Nomifensine Uptake using Positron Emission Tomography. J. Cereb.Blood Flow Metabol. 10, 307-316.

[8] Leenders KL, Salmon EP, Tyrrell P, et al. (1990) The nigrostriatal dopaminergic system assessed in vivo by positron emission tomography in healthy volunteer subjects and patients with Parkinson's disease. Arch. Neurol. 47, 1290-1298.

[9] Rinne UK, Laihinen A, Rinne JO, et al. (1990) Positron Emission

Tomography demonstrates dopamine D_2 receptor supersensitivity in the striatum of patients with early Parkinson's Disease. Movement Disorders 5, 55-59.
[10] Sawle GV, Brooks DJ, Ibanez V, Frackowiak RSJ. (1990) Striatal D_2 receptor density is inveresly proportional to dopa uptake in untreated hemi-Parkinson's disease: a positron emission tomography study. J.Neurol.Neurosurg. Psychiat. 53, 177
[11] Leenders KL, Herold S, Palmer AJ, et al. (1985) Human cerebral dopamine system measured in vivo using PET. J. Cereb. Blood Flow Metabol. 5, S157-S158
[12] Bokobza B, Ruberg M, Scatton B, Javoy-Agid F, Agid Y. (1984) [^{3}H]spiperone binding, dopamine and HVA concentrations in Parkinson's disease and supranuclear palsy. Eu. J. Pharmacol. 99, 167-175.
[13] Guttman M, Seeman P. (1986) Dopamine D_2 receptor density in parkinsonian brain is constant for duration of disease, age, and duration of L-Dopa therapy. Adv. Neurol. 45, 51-57.
[14] Leenders KL, Aquilonius SM, Bergström K, et al. (1988) Unilateral MPTP lesion in a rhesus monkey: effects on the striatal dopaminergic system measured in vivo with PET using various novel tracers. Brain Res. 445, 61-67.
[15] Fuxe K, Agnati LF, Köhler C, et al. (1981) Characterisation of normal and supersensitive dopamine receptors: Effects of ergot drugs and neuropeptides. J. Neural Transm. 51, 3-37.
[16] Quinn N. (1989) Multiple System Atrophy - the nature of the beast. J. Neurol. Nerosurg. Psychiat. Special Supplement, 78-89.
[17] Brooks DJ, Salmon EP, Mathias CJ, et al. (1990) The relationship between locomotor disability, autonomic dysfunction, and the integrity of the striatal dopaminergic system in patients with Multiple System Atrophy, Pure Autonomic Failure, and Parkinson's Disease, studied with PET. Brain 113, 1539-1552.
[18] Brooks DJ. (in press) 'PET in autonomic failure'. In R. Bannister (ed) Autonomic Failure (third edition) Oxford University Press.
[19] Steele JC, Richardson JC, Olszewski J. (1964) Progressive Supranuclear Palsy. A heterogeneous degeneration involving the brain stem, basal ganglia, and cerebellum, with vertical gaze and pseudobulbar palsy, nuchal dystonia, and dementia. Arch. Neurol. 10, 333-358.
[20] Kish SJ, Chang LJ, Mirchandani L, Shannak K, Hornykiewicz O. (1985) Progressive Supranuclear Palsy: relationship between extrapyramidal disturbances, dementia, and brain neurotransmitter markers. Ann. Neurol. 18, 530-536.
[21] Ruberg M, Javoy-Agid F, Hirsch E, et al. (1985) Dopaminergic and Cholinergic lesions in Progressive Supranuclear Palsy. Ann. Neurol. 18, 523-529.
[22] Baron JC, Maziere B, Loc'h C,et al. (1986) Loss of striatal [^{76}Br] bromospiperone binding sites demonstrated by positron emission tomography in progressive supranuclear palsy. J. Cereb. Blood Flow Metabol. 6, 131-136.
[23] Wienhard K, Coenen HH, Pawlik G, et al. (1990) PET studies of dopamine receptor distribution using [^{18}F]fluoroethylspiperone: findings in disorders related to the dopaminergic system. J. Neural Transm. 81, 195-213.
[24] Gibb WR, Luthert P, Marsden CD. (1989) Corticobasal Degeneration. Brain 112, 1171-1192.

[25] Sawle GV, Brooks DJ, Marsden CD, Frackowiak RSJ. (in press) Corticobasal Degeneration: A unique pattern of regional cortical oxygen metabolism and striatal fluorodopa uptake demonstrated by positron emission tomography. Brain.
[26] Quik M, Spokes E, MacKay A, Bannister R. (1979) Alterations in ^{3}H-spiperone binding in human caudate nucleus, substantia nigra and frontal cortex in the Shy-Drager syndrome and Parkinson's disease. J. Neurol. Sci. 43, 429-437.
[27] Rinne UK, Lönnberg P, Koskinen V. (1981) Dopamine receptors in the parkinsonian brain. J. Neural Transmission. 51, 97-106.
[28] Fuxe K, Agnati LF, Köhler C, et al. (1981) Characterisation of normal and supersensitive dopamine receptors: Effects of ergot drugs and neuropeptides. J. Neural Transm. 51, 3-37.
[29] Mishra RK, Wong YW, Varmuze SL, Tuff L. (1978) Chemical lesion and drug-induced supersensitivity and subsensitivity of caudate dopamine receptors. Life Sci. 23, 443-446.
[30] Farde L, Wiesel FA, Halldin C, Sedvall G. (1988) Central D_2-dopamine receptor occupancy in schizophrenic patients treated with antipsychotic drugs. Arch. Gen. Psych. 45, 71-76.
[31] Geraghty JJ, Jankovic J, Zetusky WJ. (1985) Association between Essential Tremor and Parkinson's Disease. Ann. Neurol. 17, 329-333.
[32] Cleeves L, Findley LJ, Koller W. (1988) Lack of association between Essential Tremor and Parkinson's Disease. Ann. Neurol. 24, 23-26.
[33] Lang AE, Kierans C, Blair RDG. (1987) Family History of Tremor in Parkinson's Disease compared with those of controls and patients with Idiopathic Dystonia. Adv. Neurol. 45, 313-316.
[34] Leenders KL, Frackowiak RSJ, Quinn N, Marsden CD. (1986) Brain energy metabolism and dopaminergic function in Huntington's Disease measured in vivo using Positron Emission Tomography. Movement Disorders 1, 69-77.
[35] Hagglund J, Aquilonius SM, Eckernas SA, et al. (1987) Dopamine receptor properties in Parkinson's Disease and Huntington's Chorea evaluated using positron emission tomography using ^{11}C-methylspiperone. Acta Neurol. Scand. 75, 87-94.
[36] Brooks DJ, Ibanez V, Playford ED, et al. (in press) Pre- and post-synaptic striatal dopaminergic function in neuroacanthocytosis: A PET study. Ann. Neurol.
[37] De Yebenes JG, Brin MF, Mena MA, et al. (1988) Neurochemical findings in neuroacanthocytosis. Movement Disorders 3, 302-312.
[38] Blin J, Baron JC, Cambon H, et al. (1989) Striatal Dopamine D_2 receptors in Tardive Dyskinesia: PET study. Neurology 39 (Supp 1), 274
[39] Andersson U, Eckernas SA, Hartvig P, et al. (1990) Striatal binding of ^{11}C-NMSP studied with Positron Emission Tomography in patients with persistent tardive dyskinesia: no evidence for altered dopamine receptor binding. J. Neural. Transmission 79, 215-226.
[40] Fletcher NA, Harding AE, Marsden CD. (1990) A genetic study of idiopathic torsion dystonia in the United Kingdom. Brain 113, 379-395.
[41] Ozelius L, Kramer PL, Moskowitz CB, et al. (1989) Human gene for torsion dystonia located on chromosome 9q32-34. Neuron 2, 1427-1434.
[42] Marsden CD, Obeso J, Zarranz JJ, Lang AE. (1985) The anatomical basis of symptomatic hemidystonia. Brain 108, 463-483.

[43] Leenders Kl, Quinn N, Frackowiak RSJ, Marsden CD. (1988) Brain dopaminergic system studied in patients with dystonia using positron emission tomography. Adv. Neurol. 50, 243-247.
[44] Playford ED, Sawle GV, Fletcher N, Marsden CD, Brooks DJ. (in press) Familial torsion dystonia: An 18F-Dopa PET study. Neurology
[45] Sawle GV, Leenders KL, Brooks DJ, et al. (in press) Dopa-responsive Dystonia: [^{18}F] Dopa Positron Emission Tomography. Ann. Neurol.
[46] Martin WRW, Stoessl AJ, Palmer M, et al. (1988) PET scanning in dystonia. Adv. Neurol. 50, 223-228.
[47] Bernheimer H, Birkmayer W, Hornykiewicz O, et al. (1973) Brain dopamine and the syndromes of Parkinson and Huntington. Clinical, morphological, and neurochemical correlations. J. Neurol. Sci. 20, 415-455.
[48] Calne DB, Langston WJ, Martin WRW, et al. (1985) Positron Emission Tomography after MPTP: Observations relating to the cause of Parkinson's Disease. Nature 317, 246-248.
[49] Calne DB, Eisen A, McGeer EG, Spencer P. (1986) Alzheimer's Disease, Parkinson's Disease, and Motor Neurone Disease: Abiotrophic interaction between ageing and environment. Lancet 1C, 1067-1070.
[50] Martin WRW, Palmer MR, Patlak CS, Calne DB. (1989) Nigrostriatal function in humans studied with positron emission tomography. Ann. Neurol. 26, 535-542.
[51] Sawle GV, Colebatch JG, Shah A, Brooks DJ, Marsden CD, Frackowiak RSJ. (1990) Striatal function in normal aging: implications for Parkinson's Disease. Ann. Neurol. 28, 799-804.
[52] McGeer PL, Itagaki S, Akiyama H, McGeer EG. (1988) Rate of cell death in Parkinsonism indicates active neuropathological process. Ann. Neurol. 24, 574-576.
[53] Duvoisin RC. Genetics of Parkinson's Disease. (1987) Adv. Neurol. 45, 307-312.
[54] Golbe LI, Di Iorio G, Bonavita V, Miller DC, Duvoisin RC. (1990) A large kindred with Autosomal Dominant Parkinson's Disease. Ann. Neurol. 27, 276-282.
[55] Johnson WG, Hodge SE, Duvoisin R. (1990) Twin-studies and the Genetics of Parkinson's disease - a reappraisal. Movement Disorders. 5, 187-194.
[56] Brooks DJ. (in press) Detection of pre-clinical Parkinson's disease with PET. Neurology
[57] Rajput AH, Rozdilsky B, Hornykiewicz O, Shannak K, Lee T, Seeman P. (1982) Reversible drug-induced parkinsonism. Clinicopathologic study Arch Neurol. 39, 644-646.

NON-HUMAN PRIMATE MODELS OF DOPAMINE SYSTEM DISORDERS : UNDERSTANDING NEURODEGENERATIVE DISEASES AND TESTING NEW THERAPEUTIC STRATEGIES

Philippe HANTRAYE

ABSTRACT. In the past decade, substantial advances have been made in our understanding of dopamine system disorders by developing working models in experimental animals, especially non-human primates. By establishing systematic correlations between the anatomical, biochemical and behavioural changes observed in these primate models and the pathological alterations specifically associated with human disorders, it has been possible to formulate new hypothesis concerning the neuropathological mechanisms possibly underlying degenerative diseases such as Parkinson's and Huntington's diseases. For example, by analyzing the location of experimental lesions of the basal ganglia in monkeys in relation with the ability of these lesions to induce abnormal movements in the animal, a hypothetical model of basal ganglia functioning was recently proposed. This model can predict the appearance of abnormal movements through the alteration of specific neural circuits. In addition, primate models of dopamine system disorders have also provided the unique opportunity of testing new therapeutic strategies such as the development of new dopamine agonist molecules or neural transplantation procedures.

1-Introduction

The development of experimental models of dopamine system disorders in non-human primates has been a very fruitful line of investigation to understand the physiopathology of the central nervous system. Thus, early studies conducted in monkeys with the aim of reproducing the symptomatology of Parkinson's disease (PD) by lesioning the substantia nigra pars compacta (SNpc) showed that it was not possible to obtain a frank parkinsonian syndrome with, in particular a typical resting tremor, after nearly complete destruction of the dopamine neurons of the SNpc. Therefore these studies have suggested that a more widespread neuronal cell death should occur in PD patients in order to explain all aspects of their symptomatology. In a same way, electrolytic lesions of the caudate-putamen designed to reproduce the striatal degeneration observed in Huntington's disease (HD) showed that even severe striatal lesions were not able to induce typical choreiform movements in experimental monkeys.

Several years ago, the use of meperidine derivatives and excitatory amino acids as selective lesioning tools offered the possibility of killing a given population of neurons in a defined brain region. Using such denervating tools, it became theoretically possible to better understand the role played by different neurotransmitter systems in the pathogenesis of degenerative diseases such as PD or HD. Further, it gave the opportunity of testing, in

J. C. Baron et al. (eds.), Brain Dopaminergic Systems: Imaging with Positron Tomography, 135–146.

experimental animals, working hypotheses formulated by clinicians to explain the symptomatology observed in patients and to evaluate the potential of new therapeutic strategies.

In the last few years, we and other groups introduced the use of non-invasive imaging techniques (Positron Emission Tomography (PET), Magnetic Resonance Imaging (MRI)) in the development and the study of experimental primate models of neurodegenerative diseases. The major interest of such non-traumatic methods is that they provide repeated measurements of various brain functions (glucidic and proteic metabolism, cerebral blood flow, neurotransmitter and neuroreceptor alterations) in the same primate, at different times after the lesion or therapeutic treatment. In addition, these techniques can be associated with other non-invasive methods (video-analysis of behavior, electrophysiology) or post-mortem studies (biochemistry, immunocytochemistry, histochemistry).

In the following, I will briefly describe various experimental primate models of dopamine system disorders, the way they were developed to improve our general comprehension of human disorders and the methodological approach that can be applied to study primate models of dopamine system disorders.

2-Primate models of Dopamine System Disorders

The main neurological disorders involving an alteration of the dopamine system and for which primate models have been developed are listed in Fig. 1. Considering the dopaminergic synapse as a reference, two different groups of disorders can be distinguished. One group consists of diseases resulting from presynaptic alterations of the dopaminergic function (loss of midbrain dopamine neurons in Parkinson's disease, striatal dopamine deficiency in Lesch-Nyhan syndrome). A second group of disorders is mainly associated with alterations of post-synaptic dopaminergic receptors (loss of striatal dopamine D2 receptors in Huntington's disease, hypersensitivity of dopamine receptors in Tardive Dyskinesia).

2.1 PRIMATE MODELS OF DOPAMINE SYSTEM DISORDERS WITH PRESYNAPTIC ALTERATIONS

2.1.1 Primate models of Parkinson's disease. In the past, electrolytic or 6-hydroxydopamine (6OHDA)-induced lesions in substantia nigra pars compacta (SNpc) in monkeys have been used as experimental models of Parkinson's disease. These studies provided information about the role of the nigrostriatal dopaminergic system (and more generally of the basal ganglia) in the regulation of motor activity, stressing the fact that the motor disorders occasioned by nigral lesions were not very pronounced (Stein, 1968 ; Delong and Georgopoulos, 1981). More recent studies confirmed that the major motor impairment resulting from lesions confined to the SNpc consists of an increase in the movement duration (bradykinesia) usually not accompanied by other typical parkinsonian symptoms such as resting tremor or rigidity (Trouche et al., 1989). On the contrary, a physiologically and radiographically controlled small lesion placed in the mesencephalic ventral tegmental area (VTA) in monkeys was shown to induce an immediate postural change on the contralateral extremity characterized by a flexed posture and the progressive development of postural tremor (Ohye, 1987). However, in typical cases, the VTA lesion in these monkeys also involved the red nucleus pars parvocellularis (RNpc) severing the cerebellothalamic pathway and a part of the nigrostriatal pathway coming from the SNpc. These observations suggest that parkinsonian tremor is related to but not the result of a single disorder in the nigrostriatal system. Other systems such as the mesolimbic and mesocortical dopaminergic pathways (Yanagisawa and Nezu, 1987); the cerebello-thalamic pathway (Ohye, 1987) or the noradrenergic system of the locus coeruleus may be involved.

PRIMATE MODELS OF DOPAMINE SYSTEM DISORDERS

NEUROLOGICAL DISORDERS	WORKING HYPOTHESES	EXPERIMENTAL MODELS
PARKINSON'S DISEASE	MASSIVE DEGENERATION OF SUBSTANTIA NIGRA	ELECTROLYTIC LESION OF A9 NEURONS 6-OHDA LESION OF A9 NEURONS
	DIFFUSE DEGENERATION OF ASCENDING DA SYSTEMS	MPTP SYSTEMIC INJECTION
LESCH-NYHAN SYNDROME	DA STRIATAL DEFICIENCY WITHOUT CELL LOSS IN SUBSTANTIA NIGRA	ELECTROLYTIC LESION OF A10 NEURONS IN YOUNG ANIMALS + D1-AGONIST ADMINISTRATION
TARDIVE DYSKINESIA	HYPERSENSITIVITY OF DA RECEPTORS	CHRONIC ADMINISTRATION OF DOPAMINE RECEPTOR ANTAGONISTS
HUNTINGTON'S DISEASE	LOSS OF POST-SYNAPTIC DA RECEPTORS	EXCITOTOXIC LESION OF STRIATUM

FIGURE 1

A few years ago, a new neurotoxin with high selectivity for catecholaminergic neurons was discovered. This drug, 1-methyl-1,2,3,6-tetrahydropyridine (MPTP), was shown to induce in non-human primates a parkinson-like syndrome (Burns et al. 1983), with features closely resembling the clinical, pathological and biochemical characteristics of PD. Different routes of administration were tested in order to develop bilateral (intravenous injections) or unilateral (intracarotide administrations) models (Bankiewicz et al. 1986). These models have been extensively used to test : 1) various working hypotheses concerning the key structures involved in the symptomatology of Parkinson's disease (Mitchell et al. 1985, Crossman 1987., Schneider et al. 1987, Delong et al.,1990) and 2) the efficacy as well as the potential adverse effects of new therapeutic treatments such as new dopamine agonists and neural transplantation (Clarke et al. 1987, 1988 ; Nomoto et al. 1985 ; Redmond et al. 1986). Even if the MPTP-primate model of PD is the best currently available, critical analyses of available data indicate that the replication of an actual parkinsonian syndrome in monkeys using the MPTP approach is very dependent on parameters such as the species of monkey used and the regimen of MPTP administration

2.1.2 Primate models of Lesch-Nyhan syndrome. Lesch-Nyhan syndrome (LNS) is a genetic disease characterized by an overproduction of uric acid and a central nervous system disorder consisting of mental retardation, choreoathetosis and a compulsive form of self mutilation. The movement disorders associated with this disease strongly suggest a possible involvement of the basal ganglia. However, neuropathological studies of brain material from patients suffering from LNS demonstrated no appreciable morphologic abnormality in any part of the brain. More recently, biochemical studies indicated that all biochemical markers of the function of the striatal dopaminergic terminals were decreased to 10-30 per cent of the control values (Lloyd et al., 1981). Based on these observations, a primate model of LNS was developed using surgical unilateral ventromedial tegmental lesions of the brain stem. In these monkeys, the levels of dopamine and the activity of catecholaminergic-synthesizing enzymes were reduced in the ipsilateral striatum. In some of these lesioned monkeys, administration of mixed D1-D2 dopamine agonists (apomorphine, L-Dopa) resulted in the occurrence of self-biting behaviour of the forelimb digits and spasticity of the hindlimbs, all symptoms typical of LNS. As indicated by these observations, the self-biting behaviour seems to be associated with the stimulation of central dopamine receptors (Goldstein et al., 1986, 1989) therefore confirming the possible involvement of dopamine neuronal abnormalities in LNS due to a loss of nigrostriatal and mesolimbic dopamine terminals (Lloyd et al., 1981)

2.2. PRIMATE MODELS OF DOPAMINE SYSTEM DISORDERS WITH POSTSYNAPTIC ALTERATIONS.

2.2.1 Primate models of Tardive Dyskinesia. Tardive dyskinesia occurs as a late complication of prolonged neuroleptic treatment in predisposed individuals (Casey and Gerlach, 1984). The syndrome classically involves involuntary repetitive movements in the orofacial region, with tongue protrusion and chewing motions, although limb and truncal choreoathetosis may also develop. Although the exact pathophysiology of this syndrome is unclear, dopamine receptor hypersensitivity is thought to play a primary role (Seeman 1988). The absence of animal models of spontaneous dyskinesia has limited research in this area. Although rodents have provided an efficient model for studying orofacial dyskinesia following long-term neuroleptic treatment (Waddington et al. 1983), these animals usually do not develop dyskinetic signs closely resembling the clinical syndrome of tardive dyskinesia. Another approach was to develop primate models of tardive dyskinesia. Two different ways have been tested so far. The first one consisted of studying the behavioral consequence of chronic neuroleptic treatment in young and aged monkeys. This approach has proved to be able to produced in monkeys reversible as well as irreversible tardive dyskinesia syndrome (Casey 1985, Kovacic and Domino 1982, Klawans and Rubovits 1972) with typical buccolinguo-masticatory movements. More recently, tardive dyskinesia was also described in parkinsonian MPTP-treated monkeys as a consequence of chronic L-Dopa or dopamine agonist treatment (Clarke et al 1987, 1988), thus emphasizing yet further the similarity of the MPTP model with the human disorder. The level of choreoathetoid dyskinesias was shown to be linearly dependent on the dose of dopamine agonist administered suggesting that peak-dose dyskinesias are linked to direct dopamine D-2 receptor stimulation.

2.2.2 Primate models of Huntington's disease. Several attempts have sought to produce involuntary movements in monkeys by making electrolytic lesions in the caudate-putamen (CP) complex (Richter and Hines 1938, Davis 1958). However, none was able to simulate "choreic movements" in monkeys even after administration of dopamine agonists (Sax et al.

1973), a pharmacological mean known to precipitate choreic movements in non-symptomatic persons at risk for Huntington's disease (HD). As an alternative, primate models based on striatal lesions induced by excitotoxins such as kainate (Kanazawa et al., 1986), ibotenate (Hantraye et al. 1989, Isacson et al. 1989) have been developed. Although these models can simulate to some extent the biochemical and pathological features of HD, involuntary movements similar to choreic movements could not be reproduced by the striatal excitotoxic lesions. Until now, only the combination of excitotoxic striatal lesions and administration of dopamine agonists has been able to reproduce in the same animal, the neuropathological, biochemical and behavioural deficits observed in HD striatum.

Neuropathological evaluation of the excitotoxically-lesioned striatum revealed a neurodegenerative pattern resembling HD with a marked neuronal cell depletion and a marked astrocytosis in the injected regions of the CP complex. After the initial studies that have been carried out in our laboratory using baboons (Hantraye et al 1989, 1990), the primate-model can now be used more specifically to test specific theories concerning HD. For instance, a theory that presently explains the increased initiation of movements through a caudate-putamen dependent circuitry (Albin et al. 1989), proposes that a disinhibition of the lateral globus pallidus by loss or blockade of GABA-ergic neurotransmission from the caudate-putamen complex, will result in a decreased pallidothalamic inhibition (via the subthalamic nucleus and the medial globus pallidus). This loss of inhibition of thalamic neurons would cause their efferent axons to excessively drive cerebral cortical motor command systems, through a putative excitatory action, thereby producing involuntary movements. The establishment of a good primate model of HD is a necessary step to elaborate our understanding of the symptomatology of the dyskinesias, including chorea. In particular, comparative studies between the location and size of the lesion of the caudate and putamen and the type of dyskinesias induced by dopamine-agonist drugs can further our knowledge of the striatum-dependent movement abnormalities. By making systematic sequential lesioning of the caudate-putamen complex one could also determine the relative and combined effect on behaviour of degeneration of the putamen, nucleus caudatus and accumbens. This may explain the progression of symptoms in HD, given the sequential development of neuronal degeneration within the caudate-putamen complex in HD.

3-The Development of Primate Models of Dopamine System Disorders

As suggested by the preceding comments, none of the primate models of dopamine system disorders currently available is fully satisfactory. However, primate models have proved already to be useful to test specific hypotheses concerning the causes of degenerative disorders and theories that may explain basal ganglia dysfunctions (Crossman 1987, Delong et al. 1990).

In considering the interest of primate models, it is important to point out that the validity of the model will be very dependent on the initial hypothesis to be tested and the overall experimental approach used to develop the model.

3.1 STRATEGY OF DEVELOPMENT.

A model of human neurological disorder should meet at least three criteria. First, it should reproduce in animals a similar or an equivalent syndrome to the one observed in patients. In addition, the symptomatology in the model should be sensitive to the same existing therapy as the human disorder. Second, the model has to present similar neuropathological changes as the disease itself. And finally, the appearance of the syndrome should follow a similar time-course as in the human disorder.

All these criteria almost require the development of the model in non-human primates. One major reason for this requirement emerges from comparative anatomical data that clearly suggest that the brain not only increased in size during recent primate evolution but also underwent disproportionate expansion and differentiation of particular anatomical structures such as the cerebral cortex or the neostriatum. Thus, according to the hypothesis of integrated phylogeny (Roof and Matzke, 1968), human neurological disorders may affect preferentially these anatomical systems according to the recency of their evolutionary modifications during primate and human evolution. In other words, non-human primates which possess a high phylogenic proximity with humans should be able, more likely than others, to replicate the neuroanatomical as well as the behavioural deficits encountered in human neurodegenerative disorders.

A possible strategy that can allow one to develop such primate models of neurodegenerative disease can be summarized as follow (Fig. 2). The first step is the careful analysis of available epidemiological, clinical, neurochemical and neuropathological data concerning the human disorder. This analysis will help to formulate working hypotheses concerning the possible causes and the degenerative mechanisms that may be involved in the disease process. The next step is to find a suitable experimental approach allowing the testing of the relevance of the hypothesis. After completion of the necessary in vivo and post-mortem studies, a careful comparison between the lesion-induced deficits and the neuropathology of the human disease will document the relevance of the model to the human disorder. If observations in the model are not relevant, a modification of the working hypothesis can be envisaged and a new experimental approach adapted to further refine the model.

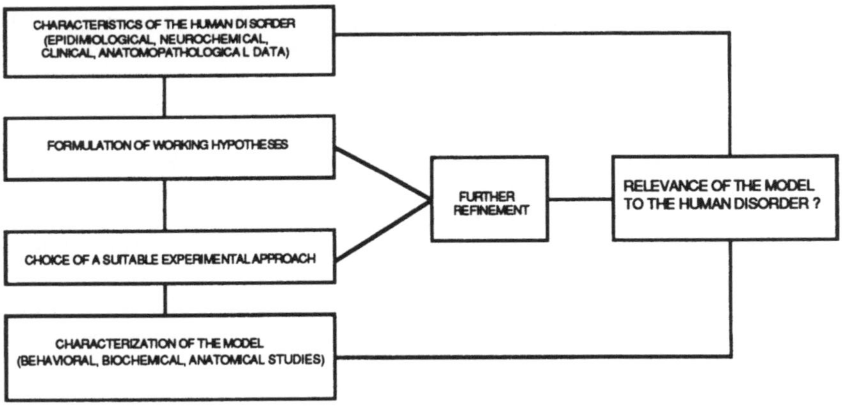

FIGURE 2

3.2 EXPERIMENTAL APPROACH .

The methodological approach used to characterize the primate model should clarify the relationships between the symptomatology observed in the living animal and the neuropathological mechanisms involved in the lesion process.

One way is to use non-invasive methods that can be performed repeatedly in vivo and to combine them with complementary in vitro and post-mortem analyses. Such multidisciplinary approach has been applied in our laboratory to study primate models of Parkinson's and Huntington's disease. Non-invasive methods included: 1)Positron Emission Tomography (PET) which provides information on neurochemical and metabolic events ; 2) Magnetic Resonance Imaging (MRI) which assess anatomy and to some extent the integrity of brain tissues and finally ; 3) behavioral evaluation of lesion-induced motor deficits using video-analysis of movements. In vitro and post-mortem methods included : 1) binding studies which can probe in vitro the regional distribution, affinity and density of specific binding sites.(this technique can provide information correlative to the observations obtained by PET, but at a cellular or sub-cellular level) ; 2) immunocytochemical and histochemical investigations.

4-Using primate models to understand degenerative diseases and test new therapeutic strategies

The development of primate models of neurodegenerative disorders must serve several purposes that can be summarized as follows :

4.1 TEST WORKING HYPOTHESES CONCERNING THE CAUSES OF NEURODEGENERATIVE DISEASES.

By mimicking in the non-human primate the typical neuropathological alterations observed in some neurological disorders, it should be possible to better understand and perhaps elucidate the neurodegenerative mechanisms underlying degenerative diseases such as Parkinson's or Huntington's disease. For example, several attempts have been conducted in the past to mimic the severe neuronal cell loss observed in the SNpc of parkinsonian patients by performing electrolytic or neurotoxic lesions (6-OHDA) of the SNpc. Comparison between clinical data and observations in non-human primates, clearly demonstrated that lesioning the SNpc only was not sufficient to produce a typical parkinsonian syndrome. Therefore, new hypotheses had tobe postulated taking into account that even if the SNpc bears the brunt of the neuronal cell loss, other brain regions also degenerate in PD. The recent discovery of a selective dopaminergic neurotoxin MPTP, allowed to refine the working hypothesis and to test the effect of a more diffuse degeneration of dopaminergic cells. In monkeys, repeated intra-venous injections of the neurotoxin under 5-8 days produced a 80-90 % destruction ofdopamine cells in the SNpc, accompanied in aged animals, by a 40-50 % dopamine cell loss in the ventral tegmental area (VTA). In terms of neuronal cell loss, this situation resembled more the situation in the human condition. However, even in animals showing both SNpc and VTA lesions it appears that there was no typical resting tremor. A further refinement of the model is clearly needed.

During the last two years we postulated as a working hypothese that chronic administration of low doses of MPTP may be able to reproduce more accurately in the monkey, the parkinsonian syndrome observed in humans. By triggering a progressive lesion of the dopamine cell bodies, chronic MPTP lesions should mimic the slowly progressing neurodegenerative process of the disease and also replicate the progression of the functional adaptative changes that should occur during ongoing lesion of the dopamine cells. Preliminary behavioral, positron emission tomography and electrophysiological observations support this hypothesis.

4.2-UNDERSTAND MECHANISMS POSSIBLY UNDERLYING DEGENERATIVE DISORDERS.

Despite our considerable knowledge of PD, a number of critical questions remains non solved. For example, the cause of neuronal cell death is unknown and the contribution of the degenerative mechanisms implicated in the progression of the disease also remains to be understood. The ability of MPTP to induce persistent parkinsonism in humans and to induce a permanent parkinsonian syndrome in monkeys has provided a clue to the cause of the idiopathic PD. For instance, the MPTP-induced lesion was shown in the primate to produce a severe and fairly selective damage to the nigro-striatal dopaminergic system. In addition, several similarities have also been noted between the MPTP primate model and the disease itself both at the biochemical and histological level. For instance, the presence of eosinophilic inclusions very similar to the typical Lewy bodies encountered in PD patients has been demonstrated in MPTP-treated monkeys. Also several lines of evidence indicate that both in the MPTP model and in PD there is a dramatic mitochondrial deficiency in the utilization of energy. Such analogies between the animal model and the human disorder at least suggest that both conditions may involve very similar neurodegenerative mechanisms.

Similarly, excitotoxic striatal lesions have previously been shown in experimental animals (including more recently non-human primates) to yield neuropathological changes remarkably similar to those of HD and have supported the hypothesis of a glutamate receptor-mediated neurotoxicity in HD. The behavioral manifestations in rodents of such striatal lesions include locomotor hyperactivity and deficits in memory and cognitive tests. However, behavioral deficits observed in the rat model of HD do not include dyskinesias or choreic movements, even following dopamine receptor agonist treatment. One major interest of developing the excitotoxic lesion model in non-human primates is illustrated by the recent discovery that unilateral excitotoxic caudate-putamen lesions in non-human primates (Papio papio, Macaca fascicularis) can elicit choreic movements after dopamine receptor agonist treatment. The relevance of such studies to pathological mechanisms involved in HD is based on the hypothesis that hyperkinesia and choreic symptoms in HD can be associated with or be mimicked by increased dopaminergic neurotransmission. In line with these observations, dopamine stimulating drugs are known to aggravate symptoms in choreic patients and have been used in some presymptomatic drug testing to detect choreic movements in persons at risk for HD.

4.3 TEST NEW THERAPEUTIC STRATEGIES.

A good primate model, well characterized in terms of biochemical, pathological and behavioral deficits, is of major interest for testing new drug therapies. Once instaured in experimental animals, the model can be used to test the beneficial as well as the adverse effects of drug treatments. A number of antiparkinsonian drugs including (+)-4-propyl-9-hydroxynaphtoxazine (PHNO) and L-Dopa have been tested using the MPTP-model and were shown to reproduce the beneficial (relief of rigidity and bradykinesia) as well as the adverse effects (L-Dopa induced dyskinesias) of equivalent therapy in PD patients (Clarke et al. 1987, 1988). Neural transplantation protocols also have been successfully tested in non-human primates and proved to alleviate, to some extent, parkinsonian symptoms in MPTP-treated monkeys. However, one particular problem of the classical MPTP-model (acute lesion in 5-8 days) developed in primates is the spontaneous behavioral recovery often observed in the 8-10 weeks following injections, rendering difficult the in vivo assessment of the drug treatment or the effect of neural transplantation. In the case of the excitotoxic striatal lesions, the model has been used recently to study dyskinesias similar to those observed in HD, their anatomical basis, diagnostic relevance, and potential therapeutic treatments to alleviate such symptoms. Preliminary results and ongoing studies indicate that neural transplantation may be a way to reduce behavioral impairments following excitotoxic striatal lesions in the primate (Isacson et al. 1989 ; Hantraye et al. in preparation).

5-Conclusion

In general, non-human primates are used as normal (control) subjects for PET studies and a majority of PET experiments conducted on them are almost entirely directed towards the development of new methods and the testing of the feasibility of studying cerebral functions in living organisms. The usefulness of PET for the in-vivo imaging of different brain functions (protein or glucose metabolism, neuroreceptors, neurotransmitter systems, oxygen consumption) is now well demonstrated. A number of biological problems can be now addressed under physiological conditions, both in humans and in monkeys. Another interest of using non-human primates in PET is to develop models of neurodegenerative diseases in order to refine existing methodological approaches for studying pathological brain functions in vivo. As PET can provide actual quantitative measurements of binding parameters or metabolic functions in vivo, a particular interest of using primate models of degenerative diseases will be to develop new imaging methods able to study the kinetics of the adaptative (plastic) mechanisms taking place after neurotoxic lesion or compensatory mechanisms brought into play after neural transplantation.

Apart from PET, other in vivo imaging techniques can also profit from primate models and the recent use of MRI in the study of neural transplantation in the primate model of HD well illustrate the potential interest of this technique for the invivo monitoring of intracerebral lesions and neural grafting. The experiments conducted in Orsay using the primate model of HD show that MRI can be very useful in addressing specific and important questions concerning the use of neural transplantation therapy for the treatment of neurodegenerative diseases(Hantraye et al. in preparation). In particular, using appropriate methodological approaches, it may be possible to answer basic questions regarding the biological consequences of intracerebral grafting procedures such as blood-brain-barrier permeability after grafting, differentiation of transplanted fetal cells into the adult host brain or graft survival. In this context, primate models will prove to be useful not only to optimize transplantation protocols, but more generally, to validate new methodological approaches applicable in clinical trials.

6-References

Albin R. L., Young A.B., Penney J.B. (1989). The functional anatomy of basal ganglia disorders. TINS, 12, 366-374.

Apicella P., Trouche E., Nieoullon A., Legallet E., Dusticier N. (1990). Motor impairments and neurochemical changes after unilateral 6-hydroxydopamine lesion of the nigrostriatal dopaminergic system in monkeys. Neuroscience, 38, 655-666.

Bankiewicz K.S., Oldfield E.H., Chiueh C.C., Doppman J.L., Jacobowitz D.M., Kopin I.J. (1986). Hemiparkinsonism in monkeys after unilateral internal carotid artery infusion of 1-methyl-4-phenyl-1,2,3,6-tetrahydropyridine (MPTP). Life Sci., 39, 7-16.

Bergman H., Wichmann T., Delong M.R. (1990). Reversal of Experimental Parkinsonism by lesions of the subthalamic nucleus. Science, 249, 1436-1438.

Burns R.S., Chiueh C.C., Markey S.P., Ebert M.H., Jacobowitz D.M., Kopin I.J. (1983). A primate model of parkinsonism : Selective destruction of dopaminergic neurons in the pars compacta of the substantia nigra by N-methyl-4-phenyl-1,2,3,6-tetrahydropyridine. Proc.Natl.Acad.Sci.USA, 80, 4546-4550.

Casey D.E., Behavioral effects of Long-term neuroleptic treatment in Cebus Monkeys (1985). In: Casey D.E., Chase , Christensen, Gerlach J. (eds) Dyskinesia, research and treatment. Psychopharmacol. (suppl. 2). Springer-Verlag, Berlin Heidelberg, pp 211-216.

Casey D.E., Gerlach J., Tardive dyskinesia : Management and new treatment. In: Stancer H.C., Garfinkel P.E., Rakoff V.M. (eds) Guidelines for the use of psychotropic drugs. Spectrum, New York, pp 183-203.

Clarke C.E., Sambrook M.A., Mitchell I.J., Crossman A.R. (1987). Levodopa-induced dyskinesia and response fluctuations in primates rendered parkinsonian with 1-methyl-4-phenyl-1,2,3,6-tetrahydropyridine (MPTP). J. Neurol. Sci., 78, 273-280.

Clarke C.E., Boyce S., Sambrook M.A., Stahl S.M., Crossman A.R. (1988). Behavioural effects of (+)-4-propyl-9-hydroxynaphtoxazine in primates rendered parkinsonian with 1-methyl-4-phenyl-1,2,3,6-tetrahydropyridine. Naunyn-Schmiedeberg's Arch.Pharmacol. 338, 35-38.

Crossman A.R. (1987). Primate models of dyskinesia : the experimental approach to the study of basal ganglia-related involuntary movement disorders. Neurosci. 21, 1-40.

Davis G.D. (1958). Caudate lesions and spontaneous locomotion in the monkey. Neurology, 8, 135-139.

Delong M.R., Georgopoulos A.P., Motor functions of the basal ganglia (1981) : in Brooks, Handbook of Physiology, vol II, pp 1017-1061, Am.Physiol.Soc., Bethesda.

Goldstein M., Kuga S., Kusano N., Meller E., Dancis J., Schwarcz R. (1986). Dopamine agonist induced self-mutilative biting behavior in monkeys with unilateral ventromedial tegmental lesions of the brainstem : Possible pharmacological model for Lesch-Nyhan syndrome. Brain Res., 367, 114-120.

Hantraye, P., Riche, D., Maziere, M., Maziere, B., Loc'h, C., and Isacson O. (1989) Anatomical, behavioural and positron emission tomography studies of unilateral excitotoxic lesions of the baboon caudate-putamen as a primate model of Huntington's disease. In Neural Mechanisms in Disorders of Movement (Crossman, A.R. and Sambrook, M.A. Eds.), J.Libbey & Co LTD, pp. 183-193.

Hantraye, P., Riche, D., Maziere, M. and Isacson, O. (1990) A primate model of Huntington's disease : behavioral and anatomical studies of unilateral excitotoxic lesions of the caudate-putamen in baboons. Exp. neurol.108, 91-105.

Isacson O., Riche D., Hantraye P., Sofroniew M.V., Maziere M. (1989). A primate model of Huntington's disease : Cross-species implantation of striatal precursor cells to the excitotoxically-lesioned baboon caudate-putamen. Exp. Brain Res. 75, 213-220.

Kanazawa I., Tanaka Y.,Cho F. (1986) 'Choreic' movement induced by unilateral kainate lesion of the striatum and L-Dopa administration in monkey. Neurosci.Lett. 71, 241-246.

Klawans H.L., Rubovits R. (1972). An experimental model of tardive dyskinesia. J. Neural Transm., 33, 235-246.

Kovacic B., Domino E.F. (1982). A monkey model of tardive dyskinesia (TD): Evidence that reversible TD may turn into irreversible TD. J. Clin. Psychopharmacol., 2, 305-307.

Lloyd K.G., Hornykiewicz O., Davidson L., Shannak K., Farley I., Goldstein M., Shibuya M., Kelley W.N., Fox I.H. (1981). Biochemical evidence of dysfunction of brain neurotransmitter in the Lesch-Nyhan syndrome. N. Engl. J. Med., 305, 1106-1111.

Mitchell I.J., Cross A.J., Sambrook M.A., Crossman A.R. (1985). Sites of the neurotoxic action of 1-methyl-4-phenyl-1,2,3,6-tetrahydropyridine in the macaque monkey include the ventral tegmental area and the locus coeruleus. Neurosci.Lett., 61, 195-200.

Nomoto M., Jenner P., Marsden C.D. (1985). The dopamine D-2 agonist LY141865, but not the D-1 agonist SKF 38393, reverses parkinsonism induced by 1-methyl-4-phenyl-1,2,3,6-tetrahydropyridine (MPTP) in the common marmoset. Neurosci. Lett. 57, 37-41.

Ohye, Neural circuits involved in Parkinsonian motor disturbance studied in Monkeys (1987). Eur.Neurol., 26, suppl.1 : 41-46.

Redmond D.E., Sladek J.R., Roth R.W., Collier T.J., Elsworth J.D., Deutch A.Y., Haber S. (1986). Fetal neuronal grafts in monkeys given methylphenyltetrahydropyridine. Lancet, i: 1125-1127.

Richter C.P., Hines M. (1938). Increased spontaneous activity produced in monkeys by brain lesions. Brain, 61, 1-16.

Roofe P.G., Matzke H.A. (1968). Introduction to the study of evolution: its relationship to neuropathology In: Minkler J. (ed) Pathology of the nervous system, Vol.1, Blakiston, New York, pp 14-22.

Sax D.S., Butters N., Tomlinson E.B., Feldman R.G. (1973). Effects of serial caudate lesions and L-DOPA administration upon the cognitive and motor behavior of monkeys. In:Advances in Neurology, Vol. 1, Huntington's chorea 1872-1972 (Barbeau A., Chase T.N., Paulson G.W., eds.), Raven Press, New York, pp 657-663.

Seeman P. (1988). Tardive dyskinesia, dopamine receptors, and neuroleptic damage to cell membranes. J. Clin. Psychopharmacol., 8, 3S-9S

Schneider J.S., Yuwiler A., Markham C.H. (1987). Selective loss of subpopulations of ventral mesencephalic dopaminergic neurons in the monkey following exposure to MPTP. Brain Res. 411, 144-150.

Stein G., The effects of lesions in the substantia nigra (1966). Brain 89: 449-478.

Trouche E., Beaubaton D., Viallet F., Apicella P., Experimental bradykinesia in the Monkey : Speed control impairments after lesion of the substantia nigra (1989). Brain Behav.Evol., 33 : 183-188.

Viallet F., Trouche E., Beaubaton D., Nieoullon A., Legallet E. (1983). Motor impairment after unilateral electrolytic lesions of the substantia nigra in baboons : Behavioral data with quantitative and kinematic analysis of a pointing movement. Brain Res., 279, 193-206.

Waddington J.L., Cross A.J., Gamble S.J. (1983). Spontaneous orofacial dyskinesia and dopaminergic function in rats after 6 months of neuroleptic treatment. Science, 220, 530-532.

Yanagisawa N., Nzu A., Pathophysiology of involuntary movements in Parkinson's disease (1987). Eur.Neurol., 26 : suppl.1 : 30-40.

THE DOPAMINE SYSTEM AND MENTAL DISORDERS: CLINICAL AND PSYCHOPHARMACOLOGICAL OVERVIEW

R. de BEAUREPAIRE

An abnormal dopamine secretion has been found or suspected in several psychiatric disorders, such as mania, depression and dementia, but it is in schizophrenia that a dopamine secretion pathology appears to be the most closely related to the disease process. The dopamine hypothesis of schizophrenia states that some dopaminergic systems, or subsystems, are hyperactive or hypersensitive in the brain of schizophrenic patients. The main support for this theory is that neuroleptics, which are dopamine blockers, improve schizophrenic symptomatology. This support has been reinforced by the finding that the affinity of neuroleptics for dopamine receptors, and specifically for the dopamine D2 receptors, directly correlates with their clinical potency (Creese et al., 1976; Seeman et al., 1976).

It is generally accepted that neuroleptics improve rapidly the acute behavioural disturbances in schizophrenic patients, and that they improve more slowly the psychotic symptoms (Casey et al., 1960; Johnstone et al., 1978). Chronic neuroleptic treatments also prevent the relapses, and this is particularly evident with depot treatments. After oral treatment withdrawal the relapses may occur within some days, but also sometimes after several weeks or months. Often the patients stop the neuroleptic treatment by themselves and they say that they feel better without it, but they practically always relapse after a variable period of time. As far as we know, the relationship between the type or the severity of the schizophrenic syndrome, or of other features such as environmental factors, and the period of time before a relapse have never been studied.

Another important point is that 10 to 20% of schizophrenic patients appear to be resistant to the neuroleptic treatment (Davis et al., 1980). However, in these cases, the use of different neuroleptics, especially atypical neuroleptics, is often effective. This raises the question as to whether neuroleptics all really have the same mechanism of action, i.e. D2 blockade. And this also leads to the idea that the

J. C. Baron et al. (eds.), Brain Dopaminergic Systems: Imaging with Positron Tomography, 147–167.

biological mechanism underlying at least some aspects of the schizophrenia syndrome may not be the unequivoqual consequence of a sole D2 dopamine receptor pathology.

Neuroleptics are also used in the treatment of mania. They improve the acute behavioural disturbances in mania, probably through a sedative effect, but they are not given chronically, the prevention of the relapses being based on lithium therapy. In psychotic depression, which is an acute delusional state, the treatment consists essentially of antidepressants, and not of neuroleptics, and the prevention is also often based on lithium therapy. Therefore, neuroleptics have at least two types of effects: one is sedative and rapid, and the other, the antipsychotic effect, develops more slowly, and appears to be specific to schizophrenia.

the different forms of schizophrenia

There are different clinical forms of schizophrenia. Today, many authors differentiate the schizophrenic syndromes according to the existence of predominant positive or negative symptoms. This can be illustrated by Crow's classification (Crow, 1985).

In this classification the type I syndrome represents acute schizophrenia with delusions, hallucinations and thought disorders, and responds well to neuroleptics. It is well known that about 30% of the acute schizophrenic episodes recover rapidly with no relapses. These acute schizophrenic episodes are called "bouffées délirantes" in France. The neuroleptic treatment can be withdrawn after a few weeks or months, the patients do not need neuroleptics any more, and in most of the cases they do not relapse. These acute schizophrenic episodes cannot be considered as schizophrenia which is a long-lasting disease. The remaining 70% (approximately) turn into chronic schizophrenia with positive symptoms but in reality, in practically all the cases, some negative symptoms are present or will appear in these patients. When they show no negative symptoms, these patients generally better correspond to other diagnostic categories, such as chronic mania, paranoia, or to the French diagnostic category of "psychose hallucinatoire chronique" (chronic hallucinatory psychosis). Consequently, only very few patients, if any, can be considered as pure type I schizophrenics.

The type II syndrome is characterized by a predominance of negative symptoms. But this does not mean that there are no positive symptoms in schizophrenics showing a type II syndrome. Delusions, hallucinations and thought disorders are the core symptoms of schizophrenia. And patients without any of these symptoms can hardly be classified as schizophrenics.

Therefore, the great majority of schizophrenic patients, if not all, simultaneously show symptoms of the type I and type II syndromes. Thus, in the view of a unitary, or of a dynamic, conception of mental diseases it may not be appropriate to insist too much on the separation of the two syndromes, which are probably indissociable, being only the two poles of a unique syndrome, namely the schizophrenia syndrome.

Crow says that the response to neuroleptics is good in the type I and poor in the type II. The reality is that the response is much more spectacular in type I than in type II, essentially because the positive symptoms are more spectacular in type I than in type II. But it is probably uneasy to sustain that the response is poor in type II, because as long as these patients are schizophrenics they do need neuroleptic treatment. And if they need a neuroleptic treatment, this means that they probably have some dopamine secretion pathology.

the autoreceptor strategy

Possible evidences of a dysfunction of the dopaminergic systems in patients with a type II syndrome are the beneficial effect of dopamine agonists (Gerlach & Lühdorf, 1976, but the patients in this study were neuroleptic-treated), of usual neuroleptic treatment (Goldberg et al., 1967), and frequently also, the effectiveness of low doses of certain neuroleptics on the negative symptoms. Amisulpride, sulpiride, pimozide and some other neuroleptics have an antiproductive effect at high doses, and a disinhibitory effect at low doses (Petit et al., 1987; Boyer et al., 1988). Disinhibitory means that the patients become more alert and active. A proposed explanation for these effects is based on the autoreceptor hypothesis which states that high doses of neuroleptics block all the D2 receptors including the post-synaptic ones and therefore have a sedative effect, but low doses of neuroleptics predominantly block the presynaptic receptors and the consequence of this presynaptic blockade is an increase in dopamine secretion which may explain the disinhibitory effect (Ungerstedt et al., 1985).

However, this explanation cannot be completely accepted because neuroleptics which are all dopamine D2 blockers do not have all this biphasic effect, and because many patients with negative symptoms do not respond favorably to the low dose treatment, and also because it has been shown that the disinhibitory effet of some neuroleptics may be related to a non-dopaminergic effect (to an S2 serotonin blockade, for instance). Nevertheless, whatever their mechanism of action, it is clear that the treatment of negative symptoms with low doses of certain neuroleptics is often very impressive, and occurs without the reappearance of the positive psychotic symptoms, so that the patients are disinhibited and not psychotic.

A long time before being applied to neuroleptics, this autoreceptor strategy was tested with dopamine agonists such as L.DOPA, apomorphine and bromocriptine in the treatment of schizophrenia. In these cases, the strategy was the same as that with neuroleptics, but with opposite effects: here the low doses were supposed to decrease the secretion of dopamine.

After the first trials, it appeared that the effects of dopamine agonists depended on many factors such as the dose, the length of treatment, the concomitant prescription of neuroleptics, and the subtype of schizophrenia. Later, the type of study (controlled or not controlled) appeared to be possibly the most important factor, since the good results of the first studies which were open studies have not been confirmed by more recent controlled studies. For example, Ferrier et al. in 1984, Tamminga et al. and Syvälahti et al. in 1986 in controlled studies, found no consistent effect with apomorphine, and Gattaz et al. in 1989, found only a transient effect with bromocriptine. Thus, low doses of dopamine agonists may have a transient sedative effect, possibly through the stimulation of presynaptic D2 receptors, but this effect is not long-lasting, and these compounds do not appear to have any real antipsychotic activity. This absence of antipsychotic activity probably demonstrates that the sole manipulation of dopamine secretion by an autoreceptor strategy is insufficiant to deal with the complexity of the phenomena implicated in psychosis. Furthermore, in several cases an increase in the psychotic symptoms have been described with the use of dopamine agonists, even at low doses (Angrist & Gershon, 1977; Tamminga, 1980).

A few successful trials on the treatment of mania and depression have been reported with dopamine agonists, particularly with bromocriptine (Dorr & Sathananthan, 1976; Saran & Acharya, 1977; Colonna et al., 1979), but here also the occurrence of some incidents such as agitation and thought disorders have been reported and the therapeutic effect were usually short-lived. Another aspect of the problem in these cases is that a specific role for dopamine in mania and depression (as well as in Alzheimer's disease) is not well established. The dopamine pathology in these conditions is more likely to be state-dependent than etiological as it may be in schizophrenia.

In fact, besides the therapeutic effects of neuroleptics, the ability of dopamine agonists to produce psychotic symptoms is classically one of the most important supports for an etiological role of dopamine in schizophrenia. However, the value of this support has been reduced with the discovery that several compounds, which are not dopamine agonists, are also able to produce psychotic symptoms. LSD, PCP, cannabis, steroids, anticholinergics and antidepressant drugs are some of these compounds. Indeed, in one way or another, all of them interact with dopaminergic systems. So that one can imagine that it is through an effect on dopamine that they are able to produce psychotic symptoms. But this may not always be the case. For instance, it has been shown that PCP can increase locomotion and produce stereotypies in animals depleted in catecholamines (Carlsson & Carlsson, 1989).

In conclusion of this section, it appears that drug-induced psychosis, as well as the autoreceptor strategy, cannot be considered today as reliable clinical and pharmacological support for the dopamine hypothesis of schizophrenia, which essentially rests on the antipsychotic activity of neuroleptics.

dopamine in the body fluids of schizophrenic patients

Another way has been proposed to test the validity of the dopamine hypothesis of schizophrenia, it is to explore the metabolism of dopamine by assaying dopamine and its metabolites in body fluids.

Several studies have shown a tendency to a decrease of HVA in the CSF of patients with predominantly negative symptoms and enlarged ventricles (Van Kammen et al., 1983; Nyback et al., 1983; Losonczy et al., 1986; Doran et al., 1987), or in relation to the severity of the symptoms (Pickar et al., 1990), but a consistent decrease in CSF HVA in schizophrenics compared to controls has not been reported (Sedvall et al., 1980; Pickar et al., 1990), and CSF studies may not be the best tool to study the metabolism of dopamine in the brain of schizophrenics because of the abundance of methodological problems. First, HVA concentrations may be 50 times less in the lumbar space than in the cerebral ventricles (Ebert at al., 1980). There are also controversies concerning the origin of HVA in the CSF, which may be cortical (Elsworth et al., 1987) or striatal (Wood, 1980), and besides, it is possible that a proportion of the lumbar HVA originates in the spinal cord (Wood, 1980). In addition, ventricular enlargements, which are a common feature in schizophrenic patients, may pose a difficult problem of dilution and clearance. There may also be some individual differences in HVA clearance. And finally, possibly the most important point is the behavioural state of the patient at the moment of the lumbar puncture, his state of activity and stress, which may be able to produce important variations in dopamine secretion (Breier et al., 1988).

Studies on plasma dopamine and HVA have given some consistent results concerning the effects of neuroleptic treatments. It seems that in general plasma HVA is increased in acute episodes and decreases in correlation with the efficacy of the neuroleptic treatment (Pickar et al., 1984). But the diet, age, sex, weight, circadian and seasonal variations, as well as the states of stress and activity, remain important methodological problems (see Losonczy et al., 1987, for review). Furthermore, the proportion of plasma HVA originating from the brain during a psychotic episode is a problematic and unresolved question.

Therefore, the determination of dopamine and its metabolites in the body fluids has brought some consistent data, but the number of methodological unanswered questions make these results only poorly informative about a possible etiological role of dopamine in schizophrenia.

post mortem studies of dopamine and its metabolites

More interesting results have been obtained with the study of dopaminergic systems in post mortem brain tissue of schizophrenics. Concentrations of dopamine and its metabolites in the striatum and the nucleus accumbens have not given consistent results (most of the studies report no changes in dopamine and metabolite concentrations in the nucleus accumbens).

An increase of dopamine and HVA in the amygdala was found by Reynolds in 1983. Interestingly, this increase was restricted to the left amygdala. Reynolds has repeated this finding in other series of brains, and also found that such changes do not occur in other brain regions (Reynolds, 1987).

Recently, Kolachana et al. (1990) have also found an increase of dopamine in the amygdala, but in the right amygdala, and not in the left, with an increase in DOPAC and not HVA.

An increase of dopamine has also been found in the thalamus, (Oke et al, 1988).

the status of dopamine D2 receptors in schizophrenia

Beside the study of dopamine and its metabolites, several investigators have focused their work on dopamine receptors.

Dopamine D2 receptors have been found to be increased in the brain of schizophrenics, while D1 receptors do not seem to be changed (although some controversies still exist on this last point). The increase in D2 receptors is generally attributed to the neuroleptic treatment (Clow et al., 1980). But some authors have found increased D2 receptors in the brain of drug-free schizophrenic patients (Owen et al., 1978; Lee & Seeman, 1980; Seeman et al., 1984). In the majority of the studies however, no increase of D2 receptors is found in unmedicated patients (Reynolds et al., 1981; Mackay et al., 1982; Kornhuber et al., 1989). Kornhuber et al. (1989) estimate three months to be the latency needed for the normalization of the Bmax after neuroleptic treatment withdrawal.

In neuroleptic treated patients, Reynolds et al. (1987) found an asymmetric increase of D2 receptors in the putamen, with a higher density in the right compared to the left. This asymmetry is in line with some clinical observations of patients who have a natural tendency to turn to their left (Bracha, 1989). A similar observation of an asymmetrical increase of D2 receptors in the putamen was made using a PET scanner in two schizophrenic patients by Crawley et al. (1986).

PET is another way to study the D2 receptors. With PET, some controversies exist about increased or normal D2 receptors in the striatum of drug-naive schizophrenic patients (Wong et al., 1986; Farde et al., 1987).

The status of dopamine D2 receptors in the brain of schizophrenic patients is probably one of the most interesting questions for the understanding of a possible dopaminergic etiology of schizophrenia, and we will review here the principal causes of a possible increase in D2 receptors in some dopaminergic subsystems of drug-naive schizophrenic patients. We found the following explanations:

- A primary defect of the dopamine receptor homeostasis, which could be related to an abnormal regulation of the gene expressing the dopamine receptor or a linked G protein.
- A hyperinnervation: increase in dopamine innervation by a developmental abnormality. There are often structural abnormalities in the brain of schizophrenics and it has been proposed that if some brain structures do not develop well, others could have an overdevelopment. This could concern some dopaminergic subsystems.
- Denervation hypersensibility (loss of presynaptic dopaminergic cells, as in Parkinson's disease).
- An abnormality in the dopamine receptor homeostasis secondary to a defective control mechanism of the dopaminergic systems such as a diminished inhibitory control. For example, after a lesion of the prefrontal cortex dopamine afferents in the rat there is an increase in dopamine turnover and of dopamine receptors in subcortical structures (Pycock et al., 1980).
- Limbic kindling, which increases dopamine metabolism and the number of dopamine receptors in the nucleus accumbens (Csernansky et al., 1988).
- Neuroleptic treatment. After neuroleptic withdrawal the normalization of the Bmax needs several weeks or months (Clow et al., 1980; Kornhuber et al., 1989).

These possible causes, except for the neuroleptic treatment, remain very speculative for schizophrenia since all of them are theoretical or emerging from experimental animal observations. On the other hand, curiously, none of them consider the possibility that schizophrenia could, at least in part, be a reactive psychosis, and the dopamine dysfunction a functional phenomenon. Little is known about the physiological changes of the dopamine receptors in the brain, and their adaptative modifications in relation to behavioural states and environmental factors. If the way through which neuroleptics have an antipsychotic effect is an increase in D2 receptors, one can imagine that such hypersensitivity could occur in the brain in the absence of neuroleptics, just as a physiological mechanism of defence against psychosis, for example in borderline personalities. In this way, it would not be surprising that D2 receptors are found to be normal in the majority of drug-free psychotic patients because in these patients the hypothetic functional mechanisms of defence against psychosis are more likely to be overwhelmed. But such possible functional adaptative mechanisms of dopaminergic systems in psychopathology have not yet given cause for much discussion to explain an hypothetic increase of D2 receptors in schizophrenia, probably because it remains a very speculative point of view with no consistent experimental support.

dopamine and the brain areas implicated in schizophrenia

If some dopaminergic subsystems are abnormally active or sensitive in schizophrenia, it is interesting to try to understand which system could be more specifically involved, and if this could correspond to some clinical aspects of the disease. Of particular interest are the striatum, the nucleus accumbens, other limbic structures, and the frontal cortex.

the frontal cortex

Several clinical, neuropsychological, and anatomical features support a major role for the frontal cortex in the physiopathology of schizophrenia. Clinically, similarities between the frontal syndrome and schizophrenia have been found for several symptoms, such as emotional flattening, inability to plan, and selective attention deficits (Weinberger, 1988). Cognitive defects of prefrontal type have also been characterized in schizophrenia, for instance schizophrenic patients appear to have specific inabilities on the Wisconsin card sorting test, a test evaluating abstract thinking and abilities to shift simple mental sets (Goldberg et al., 1987). Furthermore, although no consistant finding has been made with CT scan and magnetic resonance, structural abnormalities have been identified in the frontal cortex of schizophrenic patients by Benes et al. (1986), who found a lower neuronal density in layer VI of the prefrontal cortex. Cerebral blood flow appears to be diminished in the frontal cortex of schizophrenic patients (Ingvar & Franzén, 1974), and this hypofrontality has been confirmed by PET scan studies of glucose metabolism (Buchsbaum et al., 1982; Buchsbaum et al., 1984), even though some controversies still remain (Jernigan et al, 1985; Szechtman et al., 1988). In fact, it may be the specificity of hypofrontality in schizophrenia which is questionable, since such blood flow and metabolism disturbances are possibly state-dependant (Geraud et al., 1987; Warkentin et al., 1990). Some findings do not support a primary role for the frontal cortex dopaminergic system as a neural substrate for schizophrenia. For instance, the substantial dopamine receptor density in the human frontal cortex is of a D1 type, and not D2 (De Keyser et al., 1988; Hall et al., 1988), therefore the frontal cortex can hardly be considered as an important site for the antipsychotic activity of neuroleptics as has been previously suggested (Fuxe et al., 1985), and no change in the dopamine transmission has yet been found in drug-free schizophrenics (an increase in HVA found by Bacopoulos et al., in 1979, was probably drug induced). Furthermore, the poor performances of schizophrenics evidenced on the Wisconsin card sorting test could be related to a medial temporal lobe dysfunction (Weinberger, 1990), and selective attention defects related to a parietal dysfuction (Seidman, 1983; Posner et al., 1988). Therefore, there may be some structural and functional abnormalities in the frontal cortex of schizophrenic patients but it is not easy to link these abnormalities to a dopamine pathology at this site.

the striatum, pallidum and nucleus accumbens

These structures are rich in dopamine D2 receptors. Soft neurological signs, which are very likely to have a striatal origin, are present in approximately 50% of schizophrenic patients (Rogers, 1985). A decreased metabolic activity in the basal ganglia has been found in some PET scan studies of schizophrenic patients (Buschbaum et al., 1987; Resnick et al., 1988), but not in others (Wolkin et al., 1985; Szechtman et al., 1988), and a possible dysfunction of the putamen has been raised in the view of an asymmetry of D2 receptors in some patients (Crawley et al., 1986). Bogerts et al. (1985) have also reported a 20% decrease in volume of the medial part of the pallidum, and Bruton et al. (1990) have found a rather important non-specific focal pathology in the caudate and putamen in neuropathologic studies of schizophrenic brains. According to some authors, motor symptoms of schizophrenia could be related to a pathology of the pallidum (Bogerts, 1985; Stevens, 1986). The nucleus accumbens may, with other limbic areas, be one of the brain structures which is the most likely to be disturbed in schizophrenia (Stevens, 1973) because it is a dopaminergic structure at the interface between limbic and motor systems so that its major function is to be involved in the motor expression of emotional and motivational processes (Mogenson et al., 1980). This situation and function could explain some symptoms of schizophrenia such as parakinesias (Kleist, 1960), catatonia and mannerism (McKenna, 1987). Recently, Pakkenberg (1990) found a 40% to 50% reduction in the number of neurons in the nucleus accumbens. However, this finding is in contradiction with the results from Bogerts et al. (1985) who found no volumetric changes in the this structure. Additional neuropathological work is therefore needed. Neuropathological work with reference to dopamine has not given consistent results supporting the dopamine hypothesis of schizophrenia since dopamine and metabolites appear to be normal in the nucleus accumbens of schizophrenics (Farley et al., 1977; Bacopoulos et al., 1979; Kleinman et al., 1982), where curiously, several authors found an increase in norepinephrine (Farley et al., 1978; Kleinman et al., 1982). However, an increase of D2 receptors has been found in the nucleus accumbens as well as in the caudate and putamen of schizophrenic patients (Owen et al., 1978; Seeman et al., 1984). Therefore, the involvement of the nucleus accumbens in schizophrenia remains an interesting working hypothesis which would also fit with animal experimental models of dopamine receptor dysfunction secondary to defective control mechanisms, as discussed above.

the antero-medial temporal lobe

Several lines of evidence suggest an involvement of the antero-medial temporal lobe in schizophrenia. The most robust demonstrations arise from neuroradiologic investigations which are concordant to demonstrate structural abnormalities in this part of the brain in a large number of schizophrenic patients. Pneumoencephalography (Jacobi & Winkler, 1927) and computed tomography (Johnstone et al., 1976; Weinberger et al., 1979) showed substantial enlargements of the lateral ventricles and more recently, magnetic resonance studies reported a decrease in temporal lobe volume and limbic structures in schizophrenic patients (Suddath et al., 1989; DeLisi et al., 1988), but Kelsoe et al. (1988) found no difference in the volume of the hippocampus. According to several studies, the temporal lobe abnormalities are more likely to be lateralized to the left. Post mortem measurements have found a neuronal disarray in hippocampal pyramidal cells (Kovelman & Scheibel, 1984), a decreased volume (Bogerts et al., 1985; Colter et al., 1987; Falkai et al., 1988) and a thinner cortex (Brown et al., 1986) in the parahippocampal gyrus of schizophrenic patients. The medial temporal lobe structures are thought to be of major importance for the integration of emotional processes, and a defect in the abilities of the parahippocampal gyrus to gate sensory information could have negative effects on the functioning of other systems (Frith & Done, 1988). Memory impairments have been found in many schizophrenic patients (Koh et al., 1980) and such impairments, which may be attributed to patients lack of use of control strategies in encoding (Grove & Andreasen, 1985), could be related to a hippocampal or temporal lobe dysfunction. Many symptoms in schizophrenia such as hallucinations and thought disorders have some similarity to temporal lobe epilepsy symptoms and temporal lobe epileptics are more likely to develop psychosis than the general population (Slater & Beard, 1963). Abnormal electric activity has been recorded with deep electrodes in the limbic brains of schizophrenics (Heath, 1954), and event-related potential abnormalities on the lateral scalps of schizophrenics have been related to temporal lobe tissue loss (McCarley et al., 1989). There are dopamine D2 receptors in the limbic structures of the medial temporal lobe (Dubois et al., 1986), and these structures may be the privileged sites of action of the neuroleptics (Delini-Stula, 1986). As mentioned above, an asymmetric increase of dopamine and metabolites has been found in the amygdala of schizophrenic patients. The amygdala is involved in sensory gating, and an abnormal dopamine secretion in the amygdala could have symptomatic or behavioural consequences. An alternative hypothesis is that a medial temporal lobe dysfunction disrupts dopaminergic systems situated in other structures of the brain. Interestingly, it seems that lesions of the temporal lobe in the animal can produce a hypersensitivity to stress, with a concomitant increase of the dopamine turnover restricted to the ipsilateral nucleus accumbens (Weinberger, 1990). Bizarre schizophrenic behavior has been interpreted as secondary to an inability of the hippocampus to modulate the dopaminergic activity in the nucleus accumbens (Luchins, 1990) and amygdala kindling, which is a model of psychotic behavior (Stevens & Livermore, 1978), can change dopamine metabolism in the nucleus accumbens (Csernansky et al., 1988). Therefore, the medial temporal lobe appears to be a brain site of major interest in the physiopathology of schizophrenia, and a defect in the temporal lobe structure in schizophrenics is possibly at the origin of an imbalance in the ventral striatum dopaminergic system.

Several other brain structures may also be involved in the physiopathology of schizophrenia, such as the brainstem and the thalamus, but these structures do not appear to have the same importance regarding the metabolism of dopamine.

neuroleptics and the limbic system

The highest densities of dopamine D2 receptors are found in the striatum and in the nucleus accumbens, but the type and the pharmacology of D2 receptors may be different in these two structures. Two types of D2 receptors have been recently identified by molecular cloning, but they lack topographical differences (Giros et al., 1989). Possible differences in the funtional role of the D2 receptors have been shown by different topographical activity of various types of neuroleptics. For instance, many atypical neuroleptics appear to differ from classical neuroleptics in their behavioural effects and their regional (striatal versus limbic) sensitivity (Jenner & Marsden, 1984; Köhler et al., 1984), and in their electrophysiological properties (White & Wang, 1983). This raises the question of different topographical types and roles for the D2 receptors and the question of the localisation of the antipsychotic activity of neuroleptics.

The finding that some neuroleptics act preferentially out of the striatum is of great interest because these neuroleptics have a lower incidence of extrapyramidal side effects. Many substituated benzamides have such properties and these drugs are going through an important development today. These compounds are principally sulpiride, amisulpride, remoxipride, and raclopride; all of them have good antipsychotic activity and few extrapyramidal side effects. However, all substituted benzamides are not devoid of extrapyramidal effects. For instance, a very potent substituted benzamide, sultopride, produces extrapyramidal symptoms, and it seems that raclopride, which binds strongly to striatal dopamine D2 receptors, displays antipsychotic activity at low doses without extrapyramidal side effects, but extrapyramidal effects occur when the doses are increased.

The reason why many of these atypical neuroleptics have a higher affinity for the receptors situated in the limbic system than in the striatum is still unresolved today. The recent discovery and cloning of a new type of dopamine receptor, labeled D3, is of great interest because it is exclusively localized in brain limbic structures, but unfortunately neuroleptics do not appear to have a greater affinity for the D3 than for the D2 (Sokoloff et al., 1990). However, despite the problem of affinity, it remains possible that D3 receptors are more involved than the D2 in the antipsychotic activity of neuroleptics. This will be known when specific D3 antagonists are developed and tested in schizophrenic patients.

interactions of dopamine with other systems

From all the above discussion, it can be concluded that the specific action of neuroleptics on dopamine D2 receptors remains the most reliable support for the dopamine hypothesis of schizophrenia. However, dopamine receptors and dopaminergic systems interact with several other kinds of receptors and systems in the brain, and most of the neuroleptics have other effects than D2 dopamine blockade, so that it can be proposed that D2 receptors may not be directly involved in schizophrenia, and that neuroleptics could have an antipsychotic effect by acting directly or indirectly on other receptors than the D2.

For instance, many neuroleptics such as chlorpromazine, clozapine and flupentixol have a high affinity for the D1 receptors; cortical structures are rich in D1 receptors, and there are important interactions between the D1 and the D2 receptors. All together, these findings have renewed the interest for the D1 receptors in schizophrenia. But as far as we know, no selective D1 antagonist trial in schizophrenics has ever been reported, and D1 agonists do not seem to have any consistent antipsychotic effects (Davidson et al., 1990).

Several neuroleptics, such as clozapine, risperidone and ritanserin, inhibit more the serotonin S2 receptors than the D2, but it seems that the serotonin antagonism of neuroleptics is more related to disinhibitory than to antipsychotic properties of the drugs. Clozapine also binds to the serotonin S3 receptor, but the S3 receptor is unlikely to be the site of the antipsychotic action of neuroleptics since a selective S3 antagonist, zacopride, has no antipsychotic activity (Newcomer et al., 1990). Several neuroleptics also bind to the sigma receptors, but some major neuroleptics do not (Walker et al., 1990). An interesting glutamate hypothesis for the action of neuroleptics (Freed, 1989) and a glutamate theory of schizophrenia (Carlsson & Carlsson, 1990) have also been proposed, but for the moment they have not received much therapeutic, pharmacological or neuropathological confirmation.

conclusion

In conclusion of this review, it appears that schizophrenia is probably the only mental disorder in which dopamine has a major, possibly etiologic, role and that the ability of neuroleptics to treat schizophrenia and prevent the relapses remains the most reliable support for the dopamine hypothesis of the disease. There are very often structural abnormalities in the brains of schizophrenic patients, and such abnormalities could result in an imbalance in brain dopaminergic systems, but no result supports the idea that there is a damage in the dopaminergic systems themselves. On the whole, functional disorders of the dopaminergic systems may be secondary to structural brain abnormalities, but data are lacking in humans concerning functional disorders of the dopaminergic systems secondary to environmental factors, stressful events and their possible relation to psychosis in vulnerable persons.

REFERENCES

Angrist B, Gershon S (1977) Clinical response to several dopamine agonists in schizophrenic and nonschizophrenic subjects. In E Costa, GL Gessa (eds) Advances in Biochemical Psychopharmacology, Vol 16, pp. 677-680. Raven Press, New York

Bacopoulos NC, Spokes EG, Bird ED, Roth RH (1979) Antipsychotic drug action in schizophrenic patients: effects on cortical dopamine metabolism after long-term treatment. Science 205: 1405-1407

Benes FM, Davidson B, Bird ED (1986) Quantitative cytoarchitectural studies of the cerebral cortex of schizophrenics. Arch. Gen Psychiatry 43:31-35

Bogerts B (1985) Schizophrenien als Erkrankungen des limbischen Systems. In G Huber (ed) Basisstadien endogener Psychosen und das Borderline-Problem, pp. 163-179. Schattauer, Stuttgart

Bogerts B, Meertz E, Schonfeldt-Bausch R (1985) Basal ganglia and limbic system pathology in schizophrenia. Arch Gen Psychiatry 42:784-791
Boyer P, Puech A, Lecrubier Y (1988) Etude en double insu contre placebo de l'amisulpride (Solian°50) à faibles doses chez des schizophrènes purement déficitaires. Première analyse des résultats. Ann Psychiatr 3(supp):312-320
Bracha HS (1989) Is there a right hyper-dopaminergic psychosis? Schizophrenia Res 2:317-324
Breier A, Wolkowitz OM, Doran AR, Beller S, Pickar D (1988) Neurobiological effects of lumbar puncture stress in psychiatric patients and healthy volunteers. Psychiatry Res 2:187-194
Brown R, Colter N, Corsellis JAN, Crow TJ, Frith CD, Jagoe R, Johnstone EC, Marsh L (1986) Postmortem evidence of structural brain changes in schizophrenia. Differences in brain weight, temporal horn area, and parahippocampal gyrus compared with affective disorder. Arch Gen Psychiatry 43:36-42
Bruton CJ, Crow TJ, Frith CD, Johnstone EC, Owens DGC, Roberts GW (1990) Schizophrenia and the brain: a prospective clinico-neuropathological study. Psychol Med 20:285-304
Buchsbaum MS, Ingvar DH, Kessler R, Waters RN, Cappelletti J, van Kammen DP, King AC, Johnson JL, Manning RG, Flynn RW, Mann LS, Bunney WE, Jr, Sokoloff L (1982) Cerebral glucography with positron emission tomography. Arch Gen Psychiatry 39:251-259
Buchsbaum MS, DeLisi LE, Holcomb HH, Cappelletti J, King AC, Johnson J, Hazlett E, Dowling-Zimmermann S, Post RM, Morihisa JM, Carpenter W, Cohen R, Pickar D, Weinberger DR, Margolin R, Kessler RM (1984) Anteroposterior gradients in cerebral glucose use in schizophrenia and affective disorders. Arch Gen Psychiatry 41:1159-1166
Buchsbaum MS, Wu JC, DeLisi LE, Holcomb HH, Hazlett E, Cooper-Langston K, Kessler R (1987) Positron emission tomography studies of basal ganglia and somatosensory cortex neuroleptic drug effects: differences between normal controls and schizophrenic patients. Biol Psychiatry 22:479-494
Carlsson M, Carlsson A (1989) The NMDA antagonist MK-801 causes marked locomotor stimulation in monoamine-depleted mice. J Neural Transm 75:221-226
Carlsson M, Carlsson A (1990) Interactions between glutamatergic and monoaminergic systems within the basal ganglia - implications for schizophrenia and Parkinson's disease. TINS 13: 272-276
Casey JF, Bennett IF, Lindley CJ, Hollister LE, Gordon MH, Springer NN (1960) Drug therapy in schizophrenia. Arch Gen Psychiatry 2:210-220
Clow A, Theodorou A, Jenner P, Marsden CD (1980) Changes in rat striatal dopamine turnover and receptor activity during one year's neuroleptic administration. Eur J Pharmacol 63:135-144

Colonna L, Petit M, Lépine J-P (1979) Bromocriptine in affective disorders. J Aff Dis 1:173-177
Colter N, Battal S, Crow TJ, Johnstone EC, Brown R, Bruton C (1987) White matter reduction in the parahippocampal gyrus of patients with schizophrenia. Arch Gen Psychiatry 44:1023
Crawley JC, Owens DGC, Crow TJ, Poulter M, Johnstone EC, Smith T, Oldland SR, Veall N, Owen F, Zanelli GD (1986) Dopamine D2 receptors in schizophrenia studied in vivo. Lancet ii:224-225
Creese I, Burt DR, Snyder SH (1976) Dopamine receptor binding predicts clinical and pharmacological potencies of antischizophrenic drugs. Science 192:481-483
Crow TJ (1985) The two syndrome concept: origin and current status. Schizophrenia Bull 11:475-486
Csernansky JG, Mellentin J, Beauclair L, Lombrozo L (1988) Mesolimbic dopaminergic supersensitivity following electrical kindling of the amygdala. Biol Psychiatry 23:285-294
Davidson M, Harvey PD, Bergman RL, Powchik P, Losonczy MF, Davis KL (1990) Effects of the D1 agonist SKF-38393 combined with haloperidol in schizophrenic patients. Arch Gen Psychiatry 47:190-191
Davis JM, Schaffer CB, Killian GA, Kinard C, Chan C (1980) Important issues in the drug treatment of schizophrenia. Schizophrenia Bull 6:70-87
De Keyser J, Claeys A, De Backer J-P, Ebinger G, Roels F, Vauquelin G (1988) Autoradiographic localization of D1 and D2 dopamine receptors in the human brain. Neurosci Lett 91:142-147
Delini-Stula A (1986) Neuroanatomical, neuropharmacological and neurobiochemical target systems for antipsychotic activity of neuroleptics. Pharmacopsychiatry 19:134-139
DeLisi L, Dauphinais D, Gershon ES (1988) Perinatal complications and reduced size of brain limbic structures in familial schizophrenia. Schizophrenia Bull 14:185-191
Doran AR, Boronow J, Weinberger DR, Wolkowitz OM, Breier A, Pickar D (1987) Structural brain pathology in schizophrenia revisited. Neuropsychopharmacol 1:25-32
Dorr C, Sathananthan K (1976) Treatment of mania with bromocriptine. Br Med J 1:1342-1343
Dubois A, Savasta M, Curet O, Scatton B (1986) Autoradiographic distribution of the D1 agonist 3H SKF 38393 in the rat brain and spinal cord. Comparison with the distribution of D2 dopamine receptors. Neuroscience 19:125-138
Ebert MH, Kartzinel R, Cowdry RW, Goodwin FK (1980) Cerebrospinal fluid amine metabolites and the probenecid test. In JH Wood (ed) Neurobiology of Cerebrospinal Fluid, pp. 97-112. Plenum Press, New York
Elsworth JD, Leahy DJ, Roth RH Jr, Redmond D Jr (1987) Homovanillic acid concentrations in brain, CSF and plasma as indicators of central dopamine function in primates. J Neural Transm 68:51-62

Falkai P, Bogerts B, Rozumek M (1988) Limbic pathology in schizophrenia: the entorhinal region - a morphometric study. Biol Psychiatry 24:515-521
Farde L, Wiesel F-A, Hall H, Halldin C, Stone-Elander S, Sedvall G (1987) No D2 receptor increase in PET study of schizophrenia. Arch Gen Psychiatry 44:671-672
Farley IJ, Price KS, Hornykiewicz O (1977) Dopamine in the limbic regions of the human brain: normal and abnormal. In E Costa, GL Gessa (eds) Advances in Biochemical Psychopharmacology, Vol 16, pp. 57-64. Raven Press, New York
Farley IJ, Price KS, McCullough E, Deck JHN, Hordynski W, Hornykiewicz O (1978) Norepinephrine in chronic paranoid schizophrenia: above-normal levels in limbic forebrain. Science 200:456-458
Ferrier IN, Johnstone EC, Crow TJ (1984) Clinical effects of apomorphine in schizophrenia. Brit J Psychiatry 144:341-348
Freed WJ (1989) An hypothesis regarding the antipsychotic effect of neuroleptic drugs. Pharmacol Biochem Behav 32:337-345
Frith CD, Done DJ (1988) Towards a neuropsychology of schizophrenia. Brit J Psychiatry 153:437-443
Fuxe K, Agnati LF, Kalia M, Goldstein M, Andersson K, Harfstrand A (1985) Dopaminergic systems in the brain and pituitary. In E Fluckinger, EE Muller, MO Thorner (eds) Basic and Clinical Aspects of Neuroscience: The Dopaminergic System, pp. 11-25. Springer, Berlin
Gattaz WF, Rost W, Hübner CvK, Bauer K (1989) Acute and subchronic low-dose bromocriptine in haloperidol-treated schizophrenics. Biol Psychiatry 25:247-255
Geraud G, Arne-Bes MC, Guell A, Bes A (1987) Reversibility of hemodynamic hypofrontality in schizophrenia. J Cereb Blood Flow Metab 7:9-12
Gerlach J, Lühdorf K (1975) The effect of L-Dopa on young patients with simple schizophrenia, treated with neuroleptic drugs. Psychopharmacologia 44:105-110
Giros B, Sokoloff P, Martres M-P, Riou J-F, Emorine LJ, Schwartz J-C (1989) Alternative splicing directs the expression of two D2 dopamine receptor isomorphs. Nature 342:923-929
Goldberg SC, Schooler NR, Mattson N (1967) Paranoid and withdrawal symptoms in schizophrenia: differential symptom reduction over time. J Nerv Ment Dis 145:158-162
Goldberg TE, Weinberger DJ, Berman KF, Pliskin NH, Podd MH (1987) Further evidence for dementia of the prefrontal type in schizophrenia? Arch Gen Psychiatry 44:1008-1014
Grove WM, Andreasen NC (1985) Language and thinking in psychosis. Arch Gen Psychiatry 42:26-33
Hall H, Farde L, Sedvall G (1988) Human dopamine receptor subsubtypes - in vitro binding analysis using 3H-SCH 23390 and 3H-raclopride. J Neural Transm 73:7-21
Heath RG (1954) Studies in schizophrenia. Harvard University Press, Cambridge

Ingvar DH, Franzén G (1974) Abnormalities of cerebral blood flow distribution in patients with chronic schizophrenia. Acta Psychiat Scand 50:425-462
Jacobi W, Winkler H (1927) Encephalographische Studien an chronisch Schizophrenen. Arch Psychiatr Nervenkr 81:299-332
Jenner P, Marsden CD (1984) Multiple dopamine receptors in brain and the pharmacological action of substituted benzamide drugs. Acta Psychiatr Scand supp 311 69:109-123
Jernigan TL, Sargent T, III, Pfeferbaum A, Kusubov N, Stahl SM (1985) 18-fluorodeoxyglucose PET in schizophrenia. Psychiatry Res 16:317-330
Johnstone EC, Crow TJ, Frith CD, Husband J, Krel L (1976) Cerebral ventricular size and cognitive impairment in schizophrenia. Lancet ii, 924-926
Johnstone EC, Crow TJ, Frith CD, Carney MWP, Price JS (1978) Mechanism of the antipsychotic effect in the treatment of acute schizophrenia. Lancet i:848-851
Kelsoe JR, Cadet JL, Pickar D, Weinberger DR (1988) Quantitative neuroanatomy of schizophrenia. Arch Gen Psychiatry 45:533-541
Kleinman JE, Karoum F, Rosenblatt JE, Gillin JC, Hong J, Bridge TP, Zalcman S, Del Carmen R, Wyatt RJ (1982) Postmortem neurochemical studies in chronic schizophrenia. In E Usdin, I Hanin (eds) Biological Markers in Psychiatry and Neurology, pp. 67-76. Pergamon Press, Oxford/New York
Kleist K (1960) Schizophrenic symptoms and cerebral pathology. J Mental Sci 106:246-255
Koh SD, Marusarz TL, Rosen AJ (1980) Remembering of sentences by schizophrenic young adults. J Abnorm Psychol 72:240-246
Köhler C, Ogren S-O, Fuxe K (1984) Studies on the mechanism of action of substituted benzamide drugs. Acta Psychiatr Scand supp 311 69:125-137
Kolachana BS, Laruelle M, Casanova MF, Kleinman JE (1990) Postmortem study of dopamine and its metabolites in bilateral amygdalas of schizophrenics, cocaine addicts and controls. Soc Neurosci Abstr 16, p.1350
Kornhuber J, Riederer P, Reynolds GP, Beckmann H, Jellinger K, Gabriel E (1989) 3H-spiperone binding sites in post-mortem brains from schizophrenic patients: relationship to neuroleptic drug treatment, abnormal movements, and positive symptoms. J Neural Transm 75:1-10
Kovelman JA, Scheibel AB (1984) A neurohistological correlate of schizophrenia. Biol Psychiatry 19:1601-1621
Lee T, Seeman P (1980) Elevation of brain neuroleptics/dopamine receptors in schizophrenia. Am J Psychiatry 137:191-197
Losonczy MF, Song IS, Mohs RC, Mathe AA, Davis BM, Davidson M, Davis KL (1986) Correlates of lateral ventricle size in chronic schizophrenia. II: biological correlates. Am J Psychiatry 143:1113-1118

Losonczy MF, Davidson M, Davis KL (1987) The dopamine hypothesis of schizophrenia. In HY Meltzer (ed) Psychopharmacology: The Third Generation of Progress, pp. 715-726. Raven Press, New York

Luchins DJ (1990) A possible role of hippocampal dysfunction in schizophrenic symptomatology. Biol Psychiatry 28:87-91

Mackay AVP, Iversen LL, Rossor M, Spokes E, Bird E, Arregui A, Creese I, Snyder SH (1982) Increased brain dopamine receptors in schizophrenia. Arch Gen Psychiatry 39:991-997

McCarley RW, Faux SF, Shenton M, LeMay M, Cane M, Ballinger R, Duffy FH (1989) CT abnormalities in schizophrenia: a preliminary study of their correlations with P300/P200 electrophysiological features and positive/negative symptoms. Arch Gen Psychiatry 46:698-708

McKenna PJ (1987) Pathology, phenomenology and the dopamine hypothesis of schizophrenia. Brit J Psychiatry 151:288-301

Mogenson GJ, Jones DL, Yim CY (1980) From motivation to action: functional interface between the limbic system and the motor system. Prog Neurobiol 14:69-97

Newcomer JW, Faustman WO, Roth B, Bierley RA, Moses JA, Csernansky JG (1990) Zacopride in schizophrenia: a single blind 5HT-3 antagonist trial. Soc Neurosci Abstr p.752

Nyback H, Berggren BM, Hindmarsh T, Sedvall G, Wiesel FA (1983) Cerebroventricular size and cerebrospinal fluid monoamine metabolites in schizophrenic patients and healthy volunteers. Psychiatry Res 9:301-308

Oke AF, Adams RN, Winblad B, Von Knorring L (1988) Elevated dopamine/norepinephrine ratios in the thalami of schizophrenic brains. Biol Psychiatry 24:79-82

Owen F, Crow TJ, Poulter M, Cross AJ, Longden A, Riley GJ (1978) Increased dopamine-receptor sensitivity in schizophrenia. Lancet ii;223-225

Pakkenberg B (1990) Pronounced reduction of total neuron number in mediodorsal thalamic nucleus and nucleus accumbens in schizophrenics. Arch Gen Psychiatry 47:1023-1028

Petit M, Zann M, Colonna L (1987) The effect of sulpiride on negative symptoms of schizophrenia. Brit J Psychiatry 150: 270-271

Pickar D, Labarca R, Linnoila M, Roy A, Hommer D, Everett D, Paul SM (1984) Neuroleptic-induced decrease in plasma homovanilic acid in schizophrenic patients. Science 225:954-957

Pickar D, Breier A, Hsiao JK, Doran AR, Wolkowitz OM, Pato CN, Konicki PE, Potter WZ (1990) Cerebrospinal fluid and plasma monoamine metabolites and their relation to psychosis. Arch Gen Psychiatry 47:641-648

Posner MI, Early TS, Reiman E, Pardo PJ, Dhawan M (1988) Asymmetries in hemispheric control of attention in schizophrenia. Arch Gen Psychiatry 45:814-821

Pycock CJ, Kerwin RW, Carter CJ (1980) Effect of lesion of cortical dopamine terminals on subcortical dopamine in rats. Nature 286:74-77

Resnick SM, Gur RE, Alavi A, Gur RC, Reivich M (1988) Positron emission tomography and subcortical glucose metabolism in schizophrenia. Psychiatry Res 24:1-11

Reynolds GP (1983) Increased concentrations and lateral asymmetry of amygdala dopamine in schizophrenia. Nature 305:527-529

Reynolds GP (1987) Postmortem neurochemical studies in schizophrenia. In H Haefner, WF Gattaz, W Janzarik (eds) Search for the Causes of Schizophrenia, pp. 236-240. Springer, Heidelberg

Reynolds GP, Riederer P, Jellinger K, Gabriel E (1981) Dopamine receptors and schizophrenia: drug effect or illness? Neuropharmacology 20:1319-1320

Reynolds GP, Czudek C, Bzowej N, Seeman P (1987) Dopamine receptor asymmetry in schizophrenia. Lancet i, 979

Rogers D (1985) The motor disorders of severe psychiatric illness: a conflict of paradigms. Brit J Psychiatry 147:221-232

Saran BM, Acharya S (1977) Bromocriptine in treating mania. Am J Psychiatry 134:702-703

Sedvall GC, Wode-Helgodt B (1980) Aberrant monoamine metabolite levels in CSF and family history of schizophrenia. Arch Gen Psychiatry 37:1113-1116

Seeman P, Lee T, Chau-Wong M, Wong K (1976) Antipsychotic drug doses and neuroleptic/dopamine receptors. Nature 261:717-719

Seeman P, Ulpian C, Bergeron C, Riederer P, Jellinger K, Gabriel E, Reynolds GP, Tourtellotte WW (1984) Bimodal distr-distribution of dopamine receptor densities in brains of schizophrenics. Science 225:728-731

Seidman LJ (1983) Schizophrenia and brain dysfunction: an integration of recent neurodiagnostic findings. Psychol Bull 94: 195-238

Sokoloff P, Giros B, Martres M-P, Bouthenet M-L, Schwartz J-C (1990) Molecular cloning and characterization of a novel dopamine receptor (D3) as a target for neuroleptics. Nature 347:146-151

Slater E, Beard AW (1963) The schizophrenia-like psychoses of epilepsy. Brit J Psychiatry 109:95-150

Stevens JR (1973) An anatomy of schizophrenia? Arch Gen Psychiatry 29:177-189

Stevens JR (1986) Clinicopathologic correlations in schizophrenia. Arch Gen Psychiatry 43:715-716

Stevens JR, Livermore A (1978) Kindling of the mesolimbic dopamine systems. Animal model of psychosis. Neurology 28:36-46

Suddath RL, Casanova MF, Goldberg TE, Daniel DG, Kelsoe JR, Weinberger DR (1989) Temporal lobe pathology in schizophrenia. Am J Psychiatry 146:464-472

Syvälahti EKG, Säkö E, Scheinin M, Pihlajamäki K, Hietala J (1986) Effects of intravenous and subcutaneous administration of apomorphine on the clinical symptoms of chronic schizophrenics. Brit J Psychiatry 148:204-208
Szechtman HJ, Nahmias C, Garnett ES, Firnau G, Brown GM, Kaplan RD, Cleghorn JM (1988) Effect of neuroleptics on altered cerebral glucose metabolism in schizophrenia. Arch Gen Psychiatry 45:523-532
Tamminga CA (1980) Antipsychotic antidyskinetic properties of ergot dopamine agonists. In M Goldstein (ed) Ergot Compounds and Brain Function: Neuroendocrine and Neuropsychiatric Aspects, pp. 397-403. Raven Press, New York
Tamminga CA, Gotts MD, Thaker GK, Alphs LD, Foster NL (1986) Dopamine agonist treatment of schizophrenia with N-propylnorapomorphine. Arch Gen Psychiatry 43:398-402
Ungerstedt U, Herrera-Marschitz M, Sharp T, Ståhle L, Tossmann U, Zettreström T (1985) Caractérisation pharmacologique du dogmatil: effets pré et postsynaptiques sur les récepteurs dopaminergiques. Sem Hôp Paris 61:1283-1287
Van Kammen DP, Mann LS, Sternberg DE, Scheinin M, Ninan PT, Marder SR, Van Kammen W, Rieder RO, Linnoila M (1983) Dopamine-betahydroxylase activity and homovanillic acid in spinal fluid of schizophrenics with brain atrophy. Science 220:974-977
Walker JM, Bowen WD, Walker FO, Matsumoto RR, De Costa B, Rice KC (1990) Sigma receptors: biology and function. Pharmacol Rev 42:355-402
Warkentin S, Nilsson A, Risberg J, Karlson S, Flekköy K, Franzén G, Gustafson L, Rodriguez G (1990) Regional cerebral blood flow in schizophrenia: repeated studies during a psychotic episode. Psychiatry Res: Neuroimaging 35:27-38
Weinberger DR, Torrey EF, Neophytides AN, Wyatt RJ (1979) Lateral cerebral ventricular enlargement in chronic schizophrenic patients. Arch Gen Psychiatry 36:735-739
Weinberger DR (1988) Schizophrenia and the frontal lobe. TINS 11:367-370
Weinberger DR (1990) Limbic-cortical neural circuits and the pathophysiology of schizophrenia. Soc Neurosci Abstr 16, Opening Conference.
White FJ, Wang RY (1983) Differential effects of classical and atypical antipsychotic drugs on A9 and A10 dopamine neurons. Science 221:1054-1057
Wolkin A, Jaeger J, Brodie JD, Wolf AP, Fowler J, Rotrosen J, Gomez-Mont F, Cancro R (1985) Persistance of cerebral metabolic abnormalities in chronic schizophrenia as determined by positron emission tomography. Am J Psychiatry 142:564-571

Wong DF, Wagner HN, Tune LE, Dannals RF, Pearlson GD, Links JM, Tamminga CA, Broussolle EP, Ravert HT, Wilson AA, Toung JKT, Malat J, Williams JA, O'Tuama LA, Snyder SH, Kuhar MJ, Gjedde A (1986) Positron emission tomography reveals elevated D2 dopamine receptors in drug-naive schizophrenics. Science 234: 1558-1563

Wood JH (1980) Sites of origin and cerebrospinal fluid concentration gradients. In JH Wood (ed) Neurobiology of Cerebrospinal Fluid, pp. 53-62. Plenum Press, New York

D2 DOPAMINE RECEPTORS AND SCHIZOPHRENIA

J.L. MARTINOT

ABSTRACT. The dopamine hypothesis of schizophrenia postulates that an elevation of the D_2 dopamine receptor density could be part of the pathophysiology of the disease. To assess this question, in vivo studies of the D_2 receptors have been performed in drug-free schizophrenics using positron emission tomography. The majority of the studies invalidate this hypothesis. The role of the D_2 receptor blockade in the antipsychotic action of neuroleptics has also been extensively studied with positron emission tomography. The curvilinear relationship between the administered dose of neuroleptic and the in vivo D_2 receptor occupancy is now characterized. Studies of the link between the D_2 receptor occupancy and the antipsychotic effect of neuroleptics suggest that the D_2 receptor blockade is a necessary but unsufficient condition to explain this therapeutic effect.

1.INTRODUCTION

There are three main reasons for studying the D_2 dopamine receptors in schizophrenic patients.

First, the dopamine hypothesis of schizophrenia postulates that the dopaminergic pathways are hyperactive in this desease. The neuroleptics are know to block the dopamine receptors since the works of Carlsson and Lindqvist (1963), and consequentely overstimulation of dopamine receptors could be part of the aetiology of the disease. Such an overstimulation might be caused by overproduction of dopamine, or abnormal susceptibility or abnormal number of the receptors. As there is to date no compelling evidence of an increased activity of dopamine neurons either from cerebrospinal fluid studies or from assessment of post-mortem brain samples for metabolites of dopamine (Crow et al., 1984; Bowers et al., 1974; Post et al., 1975), the research is now oriented towards dopamine receptors.

J. C. Baron et al. (eds.), Brain Dopaminergic Systems: Imaging with Positron Tomography, 169–180.

Second, the demonstration that the antipsychotic potency of neuroleptics correlates with D_2 blockade, and not with D_1 receptors (Creese et al., 1976) has been considered as evidence that the neuroleptics exert their therapeutic action by decreasing the dopaminergic activity mediated by this class of receptors. Consequently abnormalities of these receptors have been hypothetized in schizophrenia. It should by noted however that the range of the average clinical dose for controlling schizophrenia has been discussed (Seeman 1977) and is also the dose at which side-effects are likely to occur.

Third, the density of the D_2 receptors has consistently been found elevated in the striata and nuclei accumbens of schizophrenic patients studied post-mortem by at least ten laboratories. However, a critical question of this serie of studies is to know whether the elevated density of dopamine D_2 receptors is associated with schizophrenia or whether it is simply induced by the neuroleptic medication taken by the patients before their death.

Seeman et al., (1987) reported a bimodal distribution of the D_2 receptor densities in the striata of schizophrenics neuroleptized before their death. They did not attributed this particular distribution to different premortem neuroleptic dosages, and concluded that it was associated with some aspect of the psychosis. These authors drew a parallel between their findings and the two-syndrome concept of schizophrenia (Seeman 1987).

Also, two studies (Owen et al., 1978; Lee et al., 1978) reported higher densities in drug-free patients. Moreover, postmortem studies of patients with Huntington's chorea have shown that patients who have been on neuroleptics in quantities apparently similar to those prescribed to some schizophrenic patients do not have increased Bmax by comparison with Huntington patients which have not had such medication (Owen et al, 1980).

However, recently studying the relationship between drug treatment and post-mortem striatal D_2 receptor densities in schizophrenia, Kornhuber et al.,(1989) reported increased densities only in patients who received neuroleptics within a three months period before death. Bmax values decreased with neuroleptic-free time before death, and patients off neuroleptics for more than 3 months before death were not significantly different from control values. These authors interpreted their results as evidence that enhanced Bmax values are entirely iatrogenic. This result is in agreement with the findings of Mackay et al (1982) who found unchanged values in drug-free schizophrenics, studied post-mortem.

2.IN VIVO STUDIES OF THE CENTRAL D2 RECEPTORS IN SCHIZOPHRENIA

2.1 Ligands and methods

Positron emission tomography (PET) allows the in vivo study of the striatal D_2 receptor density and affinity. Four ligands have been mainly used to investigate this class of receptors. The **methyspiperone** labelled with carbone 11 and the **spiperone** labelled with bromine 76 have a good affinity for the D_2 receptors, but their selectivity is incomplete due to their affinity for the serotonin $5HT_2$ receptors which are mostly located in the cortical regions. Fortunalely, brain D_2 receptors are mostly localized in the striata which are almost devoid of 5 HT_2 receptors, so that the radioactivity measured in the striata reflects the binding to the D_2 receptors plus the free ligand. The two other ligands are the **raclopride** labelled with carbone 11, and the **lisuride** labelled with bromine 76. They are highly selective for D_2 receptors as they do not have high affinity for other receptors.

Determining the free radioligand concentration in basal ganglia (i.e. the fraction of administered ligand which is not bound to the receptors) has been a problem in quantitative PET methods. In Orsay, we used the striatum to cerebellum ratio in our studies, which reposes on the assumption that, as the cerebellum is almost devoid of D_2 receptors, the radioactivity concentration mesured in the cerebellum at the so-called equilibrium state is an estimate of the free ligand in the brain. This index represents a measure of the density/affinity of the D_2 receptors. Also, Farde et al.,(1990) recently reported that, in a kinetic study with ^{11}C raclopride, the curve predicted by a three compartment model for the free concentration of the radioligand was almost similar to the level of the measured concentration in the cerebellum, confirming that the cerebellum radioactive concentration can be considered as an estimate of the free ligand concentration in the basal ganglia.

Two teams (John Hopkins' and Karolinska's) used a more sophisticated model to assess density of the D_2 receptors in schizophrenia. They used a kinetic three compartment model to directly measure both Bmax (the D_2 receptor number) and Kd of D_2 receptors. For this, they need both repeated PET scanning and veinous or arterialized blood sampling.

2.2 PET studies of the D_2 receptors in neuroleptic-naive or neuroleptic-free schizophrenics.

In a preliminary report published in 1985, Wong et al., did not find statistically different C_{11}-3-N-Methylspiperone (NMSP) binding between 13 chronic schizophrenics drug-free for at least one week (average off medication time : 7 months) and normal controls. These authors used the cerebellum ratio method and discussed their results, arguing that the difference may have fallen within the limits of the method and that the drug free-time may have been insufficient, so that persistent neuroleptic compound may have decreased the NMSP binding. Interestingly, they pointed to a trend of the ratio to decrease as a fonction of the number of days off neuroleptics. This study emphasized the necessity to study drug-naive schizophrenics or at least patients drug-free for a sufficient time.

2.3 Neuroleptic-free time necessary for studying D_2 receptors:

Based on PET studies of patients after neuroleptic withdrawal, (Farde et al., 1988, 1990; Cambon et al.,1987; Baron et al., 1989), we know that the D_2 receptors may be considered as free of neuroleptics 10 to 15 days after withdrawal.
However the D_2 receptors density may be increased due to the previous chronic neuroleptic treatment: Farde et al.,1990, reported that 8 weeks after withdrawal of sulpiride, the Bmax values, initialy higher than normal, were decreased, suggesting a down-regulation of the D_2 receptors. Also, in a post mortem study, Kornhuber et al.,(1989) found that there was no increase of the Bmax if the neuroleptic-free time interval prior to death was $\geq$ 90 days. These studies indicate that the up-regulation due to neuroleptics persists less than three months, and that patients untreated since at least 6 months can be considered as neuroleptic-naive.

2.4 In vivo studies performed:

Crawley et al.,(1986) used [^{77}Br]spiperone and single photon emission tomography to study four neuroleptic-naive and eight neuroleptic-free patients with schizophrenia. Their procedure allowed the calculation of striatum to cerebellum ratios but not Bmax values. They reported small (10 %) but significant ($p<.05$) increase in the striatal uptake of [^{77}Br]spiperone.
In 1986, in the John Hopkins PET center, Wong et al., used [^{11}C]N Methylspiperone and the three compartments model in a sophisticated procedure in order to study the D_2 receptor density in 11 normal volunteers, 10 drug-naive schizophrenics and 5 previously treated schizophrenics. These patients were chronic schizophrenics (duration of illness : 5 $\pm$ 3 years) which did not receive neuroleptics because they where either treated with psychotherapy or with medical care for physical health delusions. Most where

reluctant to accept psychotropic medications. The chronic schizophrenics' caudate D_2 receptor density was 2,5 fold higher than that of the control subjects (41.7 ± 4.6 and 16.6 ± 2.5 pmol of [^{11}C] N-Methyl Spiperone per gram, $p<0.02$) with a reduced overlap between the groups. In 1989, the same team reported (Wong et al., 1989) that this original sample of 10 drug naive patients has been extended to 18; D_2 receptors densities where still elevated (37.6 ± 19.8 pmol/g versus 16.0 ± 8.1 for the controls, n=19) although the overlap between the groups was more important. Recently, (Tune et al.,1990) this team extended the sample to 23 patients who had elevated D_2 receptor density, and suggested that the Bmax elevation could be most correlated with more chronic schizophrenia. Interestingly, these authors also pointed increased D_2 receptor density in manic-depressive illness with psychotic features, and a positive correlation between the receptor density and the degree of psychosis assessed with rating scales (Wong et al., 1989).

However, those results have not been replicated by other PET teams.

Herold et al., (1985) using the striatum-cerebellum ratio and [^{11}C]-Methylspiperone did not find a difference between 5 schizophrenics and controls, but a methodological artifact could not be excluded as the specific binding has not reached equilibrium in the scanning period, overlooking small differences.

Farde et al., (1987, 1990) used [^{11}C]raclopride and a three compartments model to measure both Bmax and Kd in 18 young, newly admitted and never neuroleptized schizophrenic patients. They found no significant differences in the putamen or the caudate nuclei when comparing patients to 20 controls subjects. Within the schizophrenic patients, Bmax in the left putamen was found significantly higher than in the right. This asymmetry was not found in the controls.

The Orsay group used [^{76}Br]Bromospiperone as a D_2 ligand, and the striatum to cerebellum ratio method. A group of 12 schizophrenics was studied, including 9 drug-naive patients and 3 patients drug-free for at least 1 year and never chronically treated. There was no difference when the whole schizophrenic group was compared to 12 sex- and age-matched controls. However, slight but significant differences were found when the patients whose symptoms had recently appeared or worsened were compared to the chronic patients whose symptoms were stable. The former had an higher striatum to cerebellum ratio than both the chronic without exacerbation patients and the controls, suggesting slight variations of the D_2 receptor densities with the course of the illness (Martinot et al., 1990).

We tried to replicate these results in a subsequent study using this time a new D_2 ligand, [^{76}Br]Bromolisuride, more

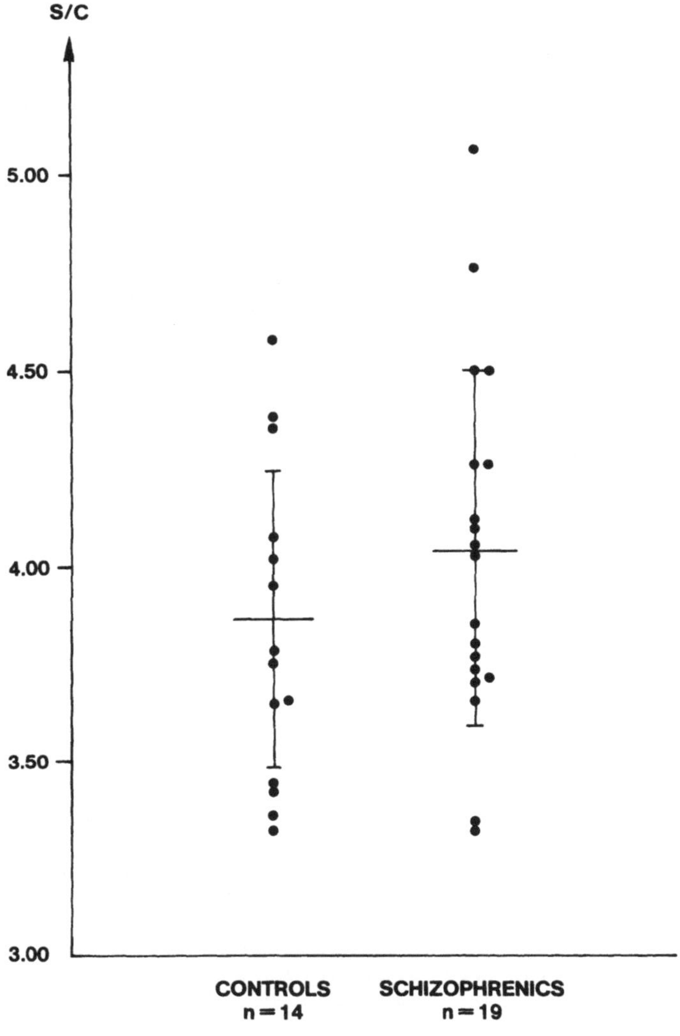

Figure 1: Striatum to Cerebellum ratio values measured with 76Br-Bromolisuride.

specific of D_2 receptors than ^{76}Br Bromospiperone. Nineteen schizophrenics (ten drug naive and nine off-neuroleptics for at least 6 months) were compared to 14 age-matched normal controls. Again, there was no difference between patients and controls in the striatum to cerebellum mean values (4.04 ± 0.46 in patients and 3.86 ± 0.38 in controls, NS, Figure 1). As in the previous study with [^{76}Br]Bromospiperone there was no relationship between the clinical types of the illness and the striatum-cerebellum values. The differences in striatum-cerebellum ratio depending on the course of the illness were not confirmed (Martinot et al.,1991).

As regards the D_2 density in the striata, it worth emphasizing that de discrepancies between J. Hopkins group's finding and the european teams' are not resulting from a situation where one study found an effect that just reached statistical significance while the others reported findings that fell short of significance. The positive finding is clear cut while the negative report are unequivocally so. A serie of differences which could contribute to the divergent results between the North american and Swedish teams have been identified in a workshop held in Montreal (Andreasen 1989).

A contribution of the Orsay group studies to the conclusions of that workshop is that the differencies in patient population probably do not explain the discrepancies: in the studies of the three teams, patients fulfilled DSM III criteria for schizophrenia, but the Hopkins patient group was older and more chronic than that of the Karolinska group. The differences observed between the chronic patients and the acute patients in the Orsay team's studies were quantitatively low, and could not be replicated in a second study; moreover, the variations of striatum-cerebellum ratios with aging in patients were not large, rendering it difficult to explain a 2 to 3 fold elevation of measured D_2 Bmax by age or course of the illness factors. Also, Orsay's team found no significant difference in D_2 receptor density between the groups of patients pooled according to the clinical types of the illness based on DSM III criteria.

As patient population's characteristics do not seems a determinant factor, the source of the mismatch should be imputed to ligand's pharmacology and modelling (which is beyond the scope of this paper). It should be emphasized than over 4 PET studies, three did not reported D2 receptor increase, with 3 different ligands. It is also noteworthy that all the studies using the striatum to cerebellum method report no, or only slight, increase of the D_2 receptor density.

3.ROLE OF THE DOPAMINE D2 RECEPTOR BLOCKADE IN THE

ANTIPSYCHOTIC ACTION OF NEUROLEPTIC DRUGS STUDIED WITH PET.

PET provides the oportunity to study in vivo the D_2 receptor blockade and its relationship to the antipsychotic effects. The relationship between the administered dose and the D2 occupancy has been studied (see Farde et al.,1988; Baron et al.,1989). A time-dependant dissociation between D2 blockade and delay of improvement or relapse of the symptoms has been emphasized. Neuroleptics block the D_2 receptors in the hours following their administration whereas the antipsychotic effect needs days to appear. After neuroleptic withdrawal, relapse of the symptoms occur after several weeks or months whereas the D_2 receptors are apparently cleared of neuroleptics in a few days.

The issue of knowing if neuroleptic nonresponder schizophrenics fail to obtain adequate DA receptor occupancy or if they do not respond to neuroleptics despite adequate occupancy has recently been resolved:

- Using [^{18}F]N-methylspiroperidol and PET, Wolkin et al., (1989) assessed the dopamine receptor occupancy in 10 schizophrenic patients before and after treatment with haloperidol. Responders and nonresponders had virtually similar indices of [^{18}F]N-methylspiroperidol uptake while treated, indicating that failure to respond was not a function of neuroleptic uptake or binding in the CNS.
- Korf et al., used ^{11}C-methyl spiperone to show that, in non responding schizophrenic patients, D_2 dopamine receptors were occupied by more than 90% (ISNIP Congress, Würzburg, june 1990).

These two studies suggest that the biodisponibility of neuroleptics at the D_2 receptor level does not necessarily account for the resistance to antipsychotic drugs. However these studies did not investigate longitudinaly the links between the D_2 blockade by neuroleptics and the antipsychotic effect.

Such a study has been undertaken in Orsay to assess these links. The striatal D_2 receptors striatum-cerebellum ratio was measured using PET and ^{76}Br-Bromolisuride in 14 schizophrenics, first untreated, and after 4 weeks receiving neuroleptics. The striatum to cerebellum ratio was also measured in 14 control subjects.

The patients received low or conventional doses of neuroleptics.

The schizophrenics (n=5) receiving low doses of energizing neuroleptics (Amisulpride 50-100 mg/day) in a double-blind way, had marked negative symptoms and few positive symptoms. Mean D_2 receptor occupancy was 20 $\pm$ 8 %. Despite this weak central D_2 receptor blockade, a moderate but significant decrease in negative symptoms was observed (Scale for the Assessment of Negative Symptoms: mean$\pm$sd total score= 86$\pm$13 before treatment and 63$\pm$27 after treatment, paired t-test= 2.65, p= 0.04), a result consistent with the hypothesis of a disinhibitory action of some neuroleptics administered in low doses. The patients treated with conventional doses (n=9) of Amisulpride, Sulpiride, Haloperidol, or Pipotiazine had "mixed" positive and negative symptoms, and the mean D2 receptor occupancy was 73 ± 18 %. Significant decreases in positive symptoms (Scale for the Assessment of Positive Symptoms: mean±sd total score= 52±32 before treatment and 23±22 after treatment, paired t-test= 2.51, df= 8, p=0.03), but also in negative symptoms (SANS total score: 86±25 before treatment and 63±13 after treatment, paired t-test=3.53, df=8, p= 0.007), were obtained with this treatment.

Before treatment, there was no significant difference in the striatal D_2 receptors striatum-cerebellum ratio between: 1/patients and controls, 2/negative and "mixed" schizophrenics, and 3/the subsequentely responder and non-responder patients. Also, after treatment, the D2 dopamine receptor occupancy by neuroleptics did not significantly differ in responder or nonresponder patients, suggesting that the central D_2 dopamine receptor blockade is a necessary, but insufficient, condition to account for the antipsychotic effect of neuroleptics. However those results do not invalidate the possibility that a relationship between D2 blockade and antipsychotic effect may exist in responder patients.

This can ben seen in perspective with the fact that D2 receptor binding of neuroleptics is the first event in a cascade of biological changes (e.g. feed-back activation of presynaptic neurons, change in the subcortical to cortical dopamine pathway balance, reversal of presynaptic activation in nigrostriatal and mesolimbic neurons, persistent increase in mesocortical activity, stabilization of presynaptic activity at a new setpoint) which are time-dependant and poorly understood. Also some neuroleptics seem to exert their action throught the newly characterized D_3 receptor.

References

Andreasen MC, Carson R, Diksic M, et al.(1988)
Workshop on schizophrenia, PET, and dopamine receptors in the human neostriatum.
Schizophrenia Bulletin 14, 471-484.

Baron JC, Martinot JL, Cambon H, et al.(1989)
Striatal dopamine receptor occupancy during and following withdrawal from neuroleptic treatment : correlative evaluation by positron emission tomography and plasma prolactin levels.

Psychopharmacology 99, 463-472.

Baron JC, Mazière B, Loc'h C, et al.(1986)
Loss of striatal 76Br-Bromospiperone binding sites demonstrated by positron tomography in progressive supranuclear palsy.
Journal of Cerebral Blood Flow and Metabolism 6 : 131-136.

Bowers MB.(1974)
Central dopamine turnover in schizophrenic syndromes.
Archives of General Psychiatry 31, 50-54.

Carlsson A, Linqvist M.(1963)
Effect of chlorpromazine or haloperidol on formation of 3-methoxy-tyramine and normetanephrine in mouse brain.
Acta Pharmacol. Toxicol. 20 : 140-144.

Crawley JCW, Crow TJ, Johnstone EC, et al.(1986)
Uptake of 77Br-Bromospiperone in the striata of schizophrenic patients and controls.
Nuclear Med. Communications 7, 599-607.

Creese I, Burt DR, Snyder SH.(1976)
Dopamine receptor binding predicts clinical and pharmacological potencies of antischizophrenic drugs.
Science 192 : 481-483.

Crow TJ, Cross AJ, Johnson A, et al.(1984)
Cathecholamines and schizophrenia : an assessment of the evidence. In : Catecholamines neuropharmacology and Central nervous system : therapeutic aspects; E. Usdin, A. Carlsson, A. Dahlström et al., (eds). New York, Alan R. Liss.

Farde L, Wiesel FA, Hall H, et al.(1987)
No D2 receptor increase in PET study of schizophrenia.
Archives of General Psychiatry 44, 671-672.

Farde L, Wiesel FA, Halldin C, et al.(1988)
Central D2 dopamine receptor occupancy in schizophrenic patients treated with antipsychotic drugs.
Archives of General Psychiatry 45, 71-76.

Farde L, Wiesel FA, Stone-Elander S, et al.(1990)
D2 dopamine receptors in neuroleptic-naive schizophrenic patients.
Archives of General Psychiatry 47, 213-219.

Herold S, Leenders KL, Turton DR, et al.(1985)
Dopamine receptor binding in schizophrenic patients as

measured with 11C-methylspiperone and PET.
Journal of Cerebral Blood Flow and Metabolism, 5 suppl. 1, S191.

Korf J, Swart JAA, Coppens JW, et al.(1990)
Cerebral dopamine receptor occupancy and quantification using radioactive spiperone and positron emission tomography : clinical and experimental studies.
Second International Symposium Imaging of the Brain in Psychiatry and Related Fields, (Abstract book).
Würzbürg June 13-16.

Kornhuber J, Riederer P, Reynolds GP, et al.(1989)
3H-spiperone binding sites in post-mortem brains from schizophrenic patients: relationship to neuroleptic drug treatment, abnormal movements and positive symptoms.
Jounal of Neural Transmission 75: 1-10.

Lee T, Seeman P, Tourtelotte WW et al.(1978)
Binding of 3H-neuroleptics and 3H-apomorphine in schizophrenic brains.
Nature 274, 897-900.

Mackay AVP, Iversen LL, Rossor M, et al.(1982)
Increased brain dopamine and dopamine receptor in schizophrenia.
Archives of General Psychiatry 39, 991-997.

Martinot JL, Peron-Magnan P, Huret JD, et al.(1990)
Striatal D2 dopaminergic receptors assessed with positron emission tomography and ^{76}Br-Bromospiperone in untreated schizophrenic patients.
American Journal of Psychiatry 147, 44-50.

Martinot JL, Paillere-Martinot ML, Loc'h C, et al.(1991)
The D2 striatal receptors estimated density in schizophrenia. A study with PET and 76Br-Bromolisuride.
British Journal of Psychiatry (in press, march 91).

Owen F., Cross AJ, Crow TJ, et al.(1978)
Increased dopamine-receptor sensitivity in schizophrenia.
Lancet 2, 223-226.

Post RM, Fink E, Carpenter WT, et al.(1975)
Cerebrospinal fluid amine metabolites in acute schizophrenia.
Archives of General Psychiatry 32, 1063-1069.

Seeman P.(1977)
Anti-schizophrenic drugs-membrane receptor sites of

action.
Biochem. Pharmacol 24 : 583-655.

Seeman P.(1987)
Dopamine receptors and the dopamine hypothesis of schizophrenia.
Synapse 1, 133-152.

Tune LE, Pearlson GD, Wong D. (1990)
Elevated D2 receptor density in 23 schizophrenics.
Schizophrenia Research 3, 29-38.

Wolkin A, Barouche F, Wolf A, et al.(1989)
Dopamine blockade and clinical response : evidence of two biological subgroups of schizophrenia.
American Journal of Psychiatry 146, 905-908.

Wong DF, Wagner HN, Dannals R, et al.(1984)
Effects of age on dopamine and serotonin receptors measured by positron emission tomography in the living human brain.
Science 226, 1393-1396.

Wong DF, Wagner HN, Pearlson G, et al.(1985)
Dopamine receptor binding of C-11-3-N-Methylspiperone in schizophrenia and bipolar disorder : a preliminary report.
psychopharmacology Bulletin 21, 595-597.

Wong DF, Wagner HN, Tune LE, et al.(1986)
Positron emission tomography reveals elevated D2 dopamine receptors in drug-naive schizophrenics.
Science 234, 1558-1563.

Wong DF, Pearlson GD, Young LT, et al.(1989)
D2 Dopamine receptors are elevated in neuropsychiatric disorders other than schizophrenia.
Journal of Cerebral Blood Flow and Metabolism 9 (suppl 1), S593.

THE ASSESSMENT OF CENTRAL D_2-DOPAMINE RECEPTOR OCCUPANCY WITH POSITRON EMISSION TOMOGRAPHY IN LONG-TERM MEDICATED SCHIZOPHRENIC PATIENTS

S. Zijlstra , J.W. Louwerens , J.A. Buddingh' , A.M.J. Paans , G. Visser , C.J. Slooff , W. Vaalburg and J. Korf .

ABSTRACT. The question was addressed whether cerebral dopamine receptors were blocked irrespective of the therapeutic response. A good response was lacking in hospitalized patients maintained on a long-term and adequate treatment with classical neuroleptics, but some of these patients improved markedly when treated with clozapine. The study concerned chronic schizophrenic patients on sustained medication. D_2-receptor occupancy was assessed by positron emission tomography using [11C]-methylspiperone ([11C]-MSP) or [18F]-fluoroethyl- spiperone ([18F]-FESP) as a ligand. Details of the procedures for the PET-ligands and scanning are given. The patient study revealed a virtually maximal receptor blockade during treatment with classical neuroleptics. These results indicate that the pathogenetic role of these receptors can be questioned in the studied chronic schizophrenic patients. Clozapine turned out to be effective as a treatment in 30-50% of the patients who were unresponsive to neuroleptic treatment. This drug probably has lower D_2-blocking properties than classical neuroleptics. PET-scanning of dopamine receptors may assist in the development of a rational treatment protocol in schizophrenia.

1. Introduction

The application of anti-psychotic drugs has dramatically changed the fate of the chronic schizophrenic patient, and thereby changed the character of the psychiatric hospitals. The anti-psychotic drugs, however, are ineffective in a substantial number psychotic patients who are often considered to be therapy resistent and require chronic hospitalization. Thus, despite the fact that the beneficial effects of antipsychotic drugs are generally accepted (Meltzer et al., 1978), during long-term use still approximately 30% of the schizophrenic patients do not respond sufficiently (Davis et al., 1986).

In vivo labeling techniques for central dopamine receptors using positron emission tomography (PET) open new perspectives (Sedvall et al., 1986). Several neuroleptics are believed to derive therapeutic effect from blocking cerebral dopamine D_2-receptors. By using tracers that have short-lived positron emitting nuclides and high affinities and selectivities for D_2-receptors, it seems possible to assess central D_2-receptor density or occupancy (Mazière et al., 1985; Farde et al., 1986). Using bromide-76 labeled bromospiperone as a ligand, Mazière and colleagues measured a 70% decrease of the specific binding in the striatum in patients who had been treated with 10 mg haloperidol per day. Farde et al. (1987;1988a,b,c) found by using [11C]-raclopride as ligand, an occupancy of approximately 80% in patients treated with a variety of neuroleptics. In a few patients D_2-receptor occupancy was related to the therapeutic effect (Farde et al., 1987). D_2-

J. C. Baron et al. (eds.), Brain Dopaminergic Systems: Imaging with Positron Tomography, 181–189.

dopamine receptor occupancy was defined as the percentual reduction of the specific [11C]-raclopride binding (in the putamen) in relation to the expected binding in the absence of the drug (measured during a drugfree period or in healthy controls).

Most of the published studies are concerned with patients responding to neuroleptic treatment (e.g. Farde et al., 1987, 1988a,b,c). We studied the extent of cerebral D_2-receptor blockade in responsive and non-responsive chronic inpatients. Patients were either treated with classical neuroleptics (non-responding patients) or with clozapine, a recently re-introduced atypical neuroleptic. Clozapine has a strong therapeutic efficacy in a substantial percentage of schizophrenic patients, who are refractory to treatment with classical neuroleptics (Kane et al., 1988).

In our studies the D_2-receptors were visualized by PET using either [11C]-MSP or [18F]-FESP, essentially according to the techniques described by Burns et al. (1984) and Coenen et al.(1988), respectively. Part of the results using [11C]-MSP have already been published (Coppens et al., 1991).

2. Methods

2.1. SUBJECTS

This study was approved by the MEC of the Faculty of Medicine of the Groningen University, all patients gave written consent.

2.1.1. *[11C]-MSP PET-scanning.* Six patients, between 22 and 40 years old, two males and four females, were examined. They were diagnosed as schizophrenics, according to the DSM-III-R criteria (Am.Psych.Ass., 1987). The patients had a psychiatric history of at least 6 years, during which they had several psychotic episodes with different responses to several neuroleptics leaving strong symptoms unaffected during the last episode. Our patients corresponded rather to the type I (predominant positive symptomatology such as hallucinations, delusions, agitation, thought disorders, etc.) than to the type II (predominant negative symptomatology such as indifference, social withdrawal, blunted affect, anergia, poverty of speech etc.; Crow, 1980, 1985). Positive symptoms are generally considered to respond better to neuroleptics (Goldberg, 1985; Keefe et al., 1987). The patients were hospitalized and treated with high dosages of neuroleptics during at least 6 weeks before the assessment. Controls were 5 healthy volunteers, all men, between 26 and 43 years of age, without any psychiatric history, and not taking any psychotropic drugs.

2.1.2. *[18F]-FESP PET-scanning.* Two patients, one female and one male, treated with clozapine resp. 250 mg and 400 mg daily, were examined. They were 25 and 28 years of age. Controls were 2 healthy volunteers, both men, 24 and 31 years of age, without psychiatric history, and not taking any psychotropic drugs.

2.2. MATERIALS

Spiperone was purchased from Janssen Pharmaceuticals (Beerse, Belgium). All other chemicals and solvents (p.a. grade) were supplied by Merck (Darmstadt, FRG) and used without further purification. High-performance liquid chromatography (HPLC) was performed on a Chrompack microporasil column (25 x 7.8 mm I.D., column A) and a Waters Radial-PAK C18 column (column B), equipped with an U.V. absorption detector (254 nm) and a radioactivity detector. For purification of [18F]-FESP column A was eluted with dichloromethane - ethanol (96:4 v/v, 2 ml/min) and column B was eluted with a acetonitrile - 0.03 m KH_2PO_4 solution (60:40 v/v, 3 ml/min). For the purification of [11C]-MSP only column A was used, and eluted with a mixture of chloroform - methanol (95:5 v/v, 2 ml/min).

Non carrier added (n.c.a.) [18F]-fluoride was produced via a $^{18}O(p,n)^{18}F$ nuclear reaction in a nickel target (2 ml), containing enriched water (50%).

Carbon-11 labeled CO_2 was obtained by bombarding Nitrogen with 20 MeV protons (Vaalburg et al., 1976) and subsequently converted to [11C]-methyliodide (Marazano et al., 1977).

2.2.1. *[11C]-MSP.* [11C]-MSP was prepared by methylation of spiperone with [11C]-methyliodide (Burns et al., 1984). Under helium flow [11C]-methyliodide was transferred into a cooled (-30 C) solution of spiperone (0.5 mg, 0.00126 mmol) in freshly distilled THF (0.25 ml). To this cold solution, TBAOH (0.4 M, 25 microliter) in water was added. The reaction mixture was magnetically stirred for 3 minutes (90 °C, water bath). After cooling down the reaction mixture to room temperature the mixture was diluted with chloroform (1.5 ml) and washed with water (1 x 1.5 ml). After evaporating the organic layer, the residue was dissolved in elution solvent (chloroform/methanol, 95/5 v/v, 1.5 ml). The solution was filtered (millipore SR-filter) and injected on HPLC. The fractions containing radioactivity (retention time 16 minutes) were pooled and evaporated. To the residue ethanol (1 ml) was added and evaporated. The residue was redissolved in ethanol (1 ml) and subsequently sterilized by filtration via a millipore FG-filter. To this solution propyleneglycol (2 ml) and saline (2 ml) were added. Radiochemical yields obtained varied from 10-15% respectively, and time of preparation was approximately 60 minutes. Radiochemical purity was above 99% and specific activities of about 400 Ci/mmol.

2.2.2. *[18F]-FESP.* To the aqueous [18F]-fluoride solution kryptofix 2.2.2 (7 mg, 0.0186 mmol) and K_3PO_4 (2 mg, 0.0094 mmol) were added. The solution was evaporated to dryness under a heliumflow at 110 °C. The residue was coevaporated with anhydrous acetonitrile (3 x 0.5 ml) in an oil-bath (110 C). To the residue a solution of 1,2-bitosyloxyethane (5 mg, 0.0124 mmol) in anhydrous acetonitrile (0.5 ml) was added. The reaction vessel was sealed and heated in an oil bath (110 C, 20 minutes). After cooling down the reaction mixture to room temperature the intermediate 2-[18F]-fluorotosyloxyethane was isolated using a pre-eluted silica seppak, eluted with a hexane-diethylether mixture (4:1, 14 ml). After evaporation of the solvent the residue was dissolved in ethanol (0.5 ml) and filtered using a millipore HV-filter. After evaporating the filtrate, spiperone (3 mg, 0.0076 mmol), kryptofix 2.2.2. (6 mg, 0.016 mmol) and K_2CO_3 (2 mg, 0.0145 mmol) were added in anhydrous acetonitrile (0.8 ml). The mixture was refluxed for another 10 minutes at 110 C. After cooling down to room temperature the mixture was diluted with dichloromethane (5 ml) and washed with water (2 x 5 ml). The organic layer was dried ($MgSO_4$) and evaporated to dryness to afford a yellow oil. The product was purified and isolated via HPLC (column A). The fractions containing radioactivity (retention time 16 minutes) were pooled and evaporated. The residue was dissolved in acetonitrile (0.5 ml) and purified via HPLC (column B). The identity of the product was established by comparison with the elution HPLC profiles of identified reference material. The pooled active fractions were diluted with water (10 ml), and the product was extracted with dichloromethane (2 x 5 ml). After evaporating the organic solvent the residue was dissolved in ethanol (0.5 ml) and evaporated under reduced pressure till dryness. The residue was redissolved in a mixture of ethanol-propyleneglycol-saline (1:2:2, 5 ml). The solution was sterilized by passing through a millipore FG-filter and subsequently injected into a stervail. Radiochemical yields were 5% and time of preparation was approximately 120 minutes. Monitoring of UV absorption and radioactivity during HPLC indicated a chemical purity > 98% and specific activities of about 2000 Ci/mmol.

2.3. PET-SCANNING

2.3.1. *[11C]-MSP PET-scans.* The scans were performed with a double headed rotating uncollimated PET camera system (Paans et al., 1985), with a total acquisition time of 32 minutes.

Scanning started exactly one hour after the injection. The specific activity of the final product varied between 200 and 360 Ci/mmol, corresponding to a tracer dose between 20-50 microgram/patient.

2.3.2. *[18F]-FESP PET-scans.* For this imaging a Siemens 951 ECAT positron camera with the new advanced computer system (ACS) consisting of 2 rings of BGO block detectors with a total axial length of 10.8 cm was used. Each detector block consists of 8x8 BGO detectors and in total 8192 detectors are employed. The data acquisition and reconstruction processes are coordinated by SUN workstation with its own disk space. Via an ethernet more workstations are installed for image analysis. The operator workstation is interfaced via ethernet to the VME bus of the advanced computer system. The ACS consists of a Motorola 68020 processor, the real time sorter, extra memory and a array processor for image reconstruction. The ACS has its own disk space available via a SCSI bus on the VME bus on which the sinograms are stored. The 68020 processor also controls the gantry and the motions of gantry and bed. The reconstructed images are stored on the disk of the operator SUN workstation and for image archiving an erasable optical disk is available.
The average spatial resolution amounted to 5.0, 5.1 and 4.8 mm FWHM in respectively the X-, Y- and Z-direction in the center of the field of view. At a radius of 10 cm these numbers amounted to 5.6, 5.2 and 5.5 mm FWHM respectively. The sensitivity as measured with 20 cm diameter, 20 cm long phantom was 125,000 cps/microCi.ml. The count rate performance, with correction for dead time, showed a linear behavior up to 5 microCi/ml. A scatter fraction of 12% was measured with a cold spot phantom.

Data acquisition was performed according to the following procedure. Before injection the patient was positioned in the PET-scanner and the gantry was tilted in such a way that planes parallel to the CM-line were selected by using the laser beams in the gantry. In this position a transmission scan was made. From this scan the emission scan can be corrected afterwards for the attenuation. After this, the patient was injected with [18F]-FESP, dose up to 185 MBq. The specific activity of the final product varied between 500 - 2000 Ci/mmol, corresponding to a tracer dose between 2-8 microgram/patient. At 3 and 4 hours after injection data acquisition was performed for a period of 20 minutes. To estimate the striatal cerebellar ratio, the striatum was outlined to a size in correspondence to its anatomical size.

2.4. D_2-RECEPTOR OCCUPANCY

The occupancy of the central D_2-dopamine receptor was estimated from the relative radioactivity in the bilateral striatum and cerebellum. The ipsilateral count density observed in the striatum was divided by the count density in the ipsilateral part of the cerebellum (considered as a measure for the nonspecific binding). In this way the specific binding to the free (i.e. not blocked by the neuroleptics) D_2-receptors in the striatum was expressed as the ratio to the non specific binding in the cerebellum (Rutgers et al., 1987). The amount of D_2-receptors in the cerebellum is negligible (Martres et al., 1985; Farde et al., 1988a).

3. Results

3.1 THE [11C]-MSP PET-SCANS

In none of the 6 medicated patients striatal D_2-dopamine receptors could be discerned. This implies that the specific binding sites of the radioligand were apparently fully occupied by the antipsychotic drugs. In five healthy controls the striatum to cerebellum ratio was 2.5 to 3.2 (mean ± SEM: 2.92 ± 0.18). This is in agreement with the results of e.g. Smith et al. (1988) who used

[18]F-methylspiperone and found under similar experimental conditions a mean ratio striatum to cerebellum of 3.65 in 5 controls . In the patients the ratio was in between 0.99 and 1.16. From these results we estimated a receptor occupancy of more than 95% during classical neuroleptic treatment.

3.2. THE [18F]-FESP PET-SCANS

The prelimary results of the two patients and volunteers indicate, that during clozapine treatment the striatal cerebellar ratio is close to the striatal cerebellar ratio in volunteers. An example of these scans are shown in the following figures. The first scan shows the accumulation of [18F]-FESP in a normal volunteer. The second scan shows the accumulation in a schizophrenic patient treated with clozapine. This scan is not corrected for attenuation. Both scans are performed 3 hours after injection.

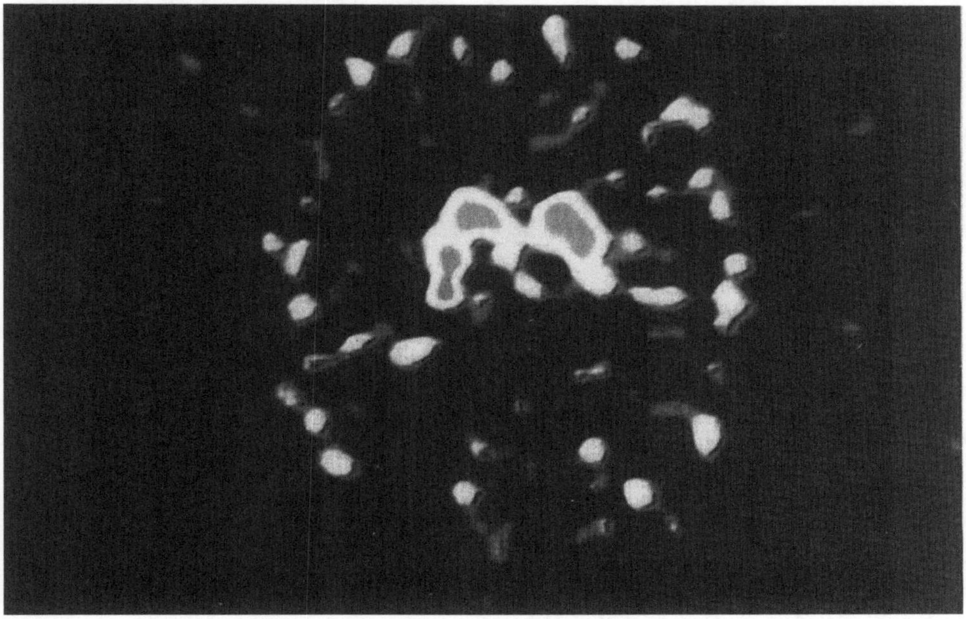

[18F]-FESP PET-scans of the brain of a normal volunteer in this study.

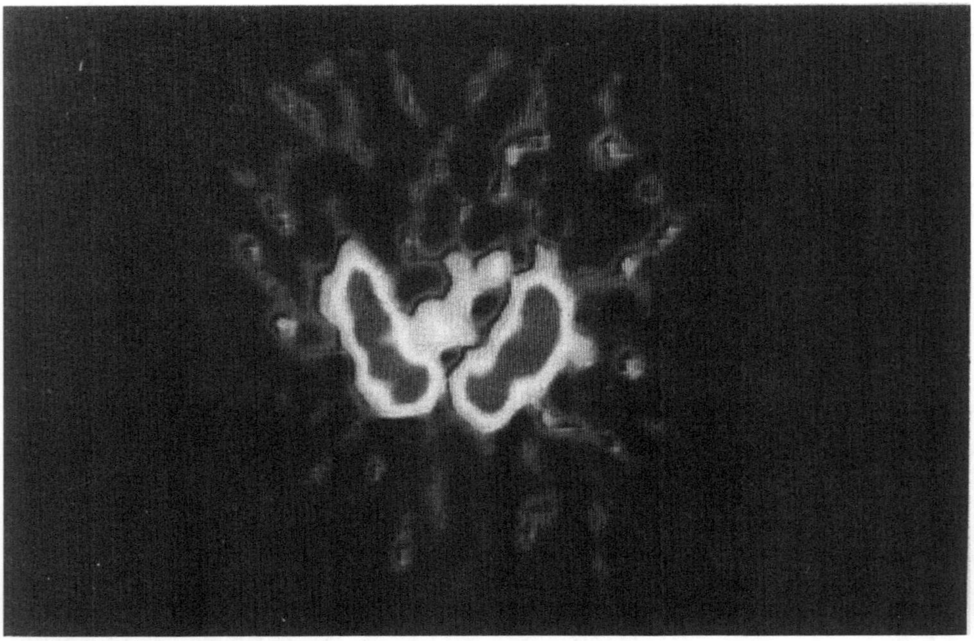

[18F]-FESP PET-scan of the brain of a patient of this study.

4. Discussion

The PET-method has been used to estimate the receptor occupancy in neuroleptic treatment. Farde et al. (1988b,1988c), using [11C]-raclopride, reported a 65 to 85% receptor occupancy, which was related to a substantial clinical benefit, expressed as a mean reduction on the brief psychiatric rating scale of 64%. We estimated that about 97% of the D_2-receptors were occupied during relatively high dose neuroleptic therapy. These estimates may be somewhat too high, because we supposed nonspecific and free ligand concentration in the studied brain regions to be equal. In addition, an instrumental error of about 10% may also contribute to the incertainty estimations (Paans et al.,1985; Rutgers et al.,1987).

Regarding the D_2-receptor blockade it does not seem meaningful to elevate the dosages of neuroleptics, or to change to another anti-dopaminergic neuroleptic treatment if achieving a better antipsychotic effect is the aim. The lack of obvious clinical response in our patients is not due to a failure of drug resorption, blood brain barrier penetration or hypermetabolism; the target (cerebral D_2-dopamine receptors) is abundantly reached. Our results indicate that it can be virtually excluded that pharmacodynamic or pharmacokinetic problems contribute to the therapy resistance of the examined patients. This conclusion is in agreement with Wolkin et al.(1989).

So the question about the significance of the central D_2-receptor blockade for the antipsychotic action remains, at least in a subgroup of schizophrenic patients. Considering other treatment regimens possible therapeutic responses may be achieved only when in addition to a blockade of the central D_2-receptors other neuroreceptors may be manipulated. This may be effected as well by addition of other drugs to neuroleptic monotherapy or with the atypical neuroleptic clozapine.

We observed that clozapine gave a far lower D_2-receptor blockade than typical neuroleptics do. These observations were obtained by using a Siemens 951 ECAT camera. Imaging of the patients, treated with typical neuroleptics, was not performed with this camera.

So the therapeutic efficacy must be attributed to additional effects on brain physiology. In a related study by Wolkin et al. (1989) it was concluded that there may exist biological subtypes of schizophrenic patients, but we suggest that also in the course of the disease a responsive patient may render into a patient no longer responding to treatment with neuroleptic monotherapy. In the past 4 out of the 6 patients have had a complete remission of the psychotic symptoms. These remissions can probably be ascribed to medication with neuroleptics and the result of central D_2-receptor blockade. Nevertheless, the symptoms did not respond to the same neuroleptics in a later stage of the disease. We suppose that some adaptional or progressive degenerative mechanism could be involved. It is not known whether such an adaptive process occurs at the receptor level.

In view of the dopamine hypothesis on schizophrenia our results substantiate the generally accepted view that during neuroleptic therapy central dopamine receptors are blocked to a major degree. On the other hand our data do not support the idea (Wong et al., 1986) that dopamine D_2-receptors are pathogenetically involved in the maintainance of the schizophrenic state in chronically affected patients.

These studies illustrate the possibilities of PET in investigating pathological mechanism underlying schizophrenia and how clinical therapeutic practice can be influenced accordingly. Development of new antipsychotic drugs can be guided by PET research, considering that D_2 blocking properties no longer exclusively predict antipsychotic effectivity. Clinical applications of ligand binding to other central receptors may contribute to the understanding which cerebral processes may or may not be involved in the lack of therapeutic responds to classical neuroleptics or to the positive effect of atypical neuroleptics, including clozapine.

Acknowledgements

This study was financially supported by Sandoz B.V. and the Netherlands Organization of Science (NWO).

5. References

American Psychiatric Association (1987): (DSMIII-R) diagnostic and statistical Manual of mental disorders (3rd edition, revised). Eds: Spitzer, R.L. and Williams, J.B.W., Washington DC, APA.

Burns, H.D., Dannals, R.F., Langstrom, B., Ravert, H.T., Zomeyom, S.E., Duelfer, T., Wong, D.F., Frost, F.F., Kuhar, M.J. and Wagner, H.N. (1984) '3-N-[11C]-methylspiperone, a ligand binding to dopamine receptors: radiochemical synthesis and biodistribution in mice', J. Nucl. Med. 25: 1222-1227.

Coenen, H.H., Wienhard, K., Stocklin, G., Laufer, P., Hebold, I., Pawlik, G. and Heiss, W.D. (1988) 'PET measurement of D_2 and S_2 receptor binding of 3-N-([18F]fluoroethyl)spiperone in baboon brain', Eur. J. Nucl.Med. 14, 80-87.

Coppens, H.J., Slooff, C.J., Paans, A.M.J., Wiegman, T., Vaalburg, W. and Korf, J. (1990) 'High central D_2-Dopamine receptor occupancy as assessed with positron emission tomography in medicated but therapy resistant schizophrenic patients', Biol. Psychiatry in press.

Crow, T.J. (1980) 'Molecular pathology of schizofrenia: more than one disease process?', Br. Med. J. 280, 66-68.

Crow, T.J. (1985) 'The two syndrome concept origins and current status', Schizophrenia Bull 11, 471.

Davis, J.M. and Andriukaitis, J. (1986) 'The natural course of schizophrenia and effective maintenance drug treatment', J. Clin. Psychopharmacol 6, 25-105.

Farde, L., Hall, H., Ehrin, E. and Sedvall, G. (1986) 'Quantitative analysis of D2 dopamine receptor binding in the living human brain by PET', Science 231, 258-261.

Farde, L., Halldin, C., Stone-Elander, S. and Sedvall, G. (1987) 'PET analysis of human dopamine receptor subtypes using [11C]-SCH 23390 and [11C]-raclopride', Psychopharmacology 92, 278-284.

Farde, L., Panli, S., Hall, H., Eriksson, L., Halldin, C., Hogberg, T., Nilsson, L., Sjogren, E. and Stone-Elander, S. (1988a) 'Stereoselective binding of [11C]-raclopride in living human brain - a search for extra striatal central D2-dopamine receptors by PET', Psychopharmacology 94, 471-478.

Farde, L., Wiesel, F.A., Halldin, C and Sedvall, G. (1988b) 'Central D_2-dopamine receptor occupancy in schizophrenic patients treated with antipsychotic drugs', Arch. Gen. Psychiat. 45, 71- 76.

Farde, L., Wiesel, F.A., Jansson, P., Uppfeldt, G., Wahlen, G. and Sedvall, G. (1988c) 'An open label trial of raclopride in acute schizophrenia, conformation of D_2-dopamine receptor accupancy by PET', Psychopharmacology 94, 1-7.

Goldberg, S.C. (1985) 'Negative and deficit symptoms in schizophrenia do respond to neuroleptics', Schizophrenia Bull. 11, 453-456.

Kane, J.M., Honigfield, G., Singer, J. and Meltze,r H.Y. (1988) 'Clozapine for the treatment-resistant schizofrenic: results of a United States multicenter trial', Psychopharmacology 99, s60-s63.

Keefe, R.S.E., Moha, R.C., Losonczy, M.F., Davidson, M., Silverman, G.M., Kendler, K.S., Horvalls, T.B., Nora, R. and Davia K.L. (1987) 'Characteristics of very poor outcome schizophrenia', Am. J. Psychiat. 144, 889-895.

Louwerens, J. W., Coppens, H.J., Korf, J., Slooff, C.J., Paans, A.M.J. and Vaalburg, W. (1990) 'On the pathogenetic role of dopaminergic and serotonergic neurotransmission in long-term hospitalized psychotic patients', Schiz. Res. 3, 52.

Marazano, C., Maziere, M., Berger, B. and Comar, D. (1977) 'Synthesis of [11C]-methyliodide and [11C]-formaldehyde', Int. J. Appl. Radiat. Isot. 28, 49.

Martres, M.P., Bouthenet, M.L., Sales, N., Sokoloff, P. and Schwartz, J.C. (1985) 'Widespread distribution of brain dopamine receptors evidenced with [125I]-iodosulpride, a highly selective ligand', Science 228, 752-754.

Maziere, B., Loch, C., Baron, J.C., Sgouzopoulos, P., Anguesnoy, N., D'antona, R. and Cambon, H. (1985) 'In vivo quantitative imaging of dopamine receptors in human brain using positron tomograph and [76Br]-bromospiperone', Eur. J. Pharmacol. 114, 267-272.

Meltzer, H.Y., Goode, D.J., Schyve, P.M., Young, M. and Fang, V.S. (1978) 'Effect of clozapine on human serum prolactin levels', Am. J. Psychiatry 136, 1550-1555.

Paans, A.M.J., Vaalburg, W. and Woldring, M.G. (1985) 'A rotating double-headed positron camera', J. Nucl. Med. 26, 1466-1471.

Rutgers, A.W.F, Lakke, J.P.W.F., Paans, A.M.J, Vaalburg, W. and Korf, J. (1987) 'Tracing of dopamine receptors in hemiparkinsonism with positron emission tomography', J. Neurol. Sci. 80, 237-247.

Sedvall, G., Farde, L., Persson, A. and Wiesel, F.A. (1986) 'Imaging of neurotransmitter receptors in the living human brain', Arch. Gen. Psychiat. 43, 995-1005.

Smith, M., Wolf, A.F., Brooke, S.D., Arnett, C.D., Barouche, F., Shine, C.Y., Fowler, J.S., Ranell, J.A.G., MacGregor, R.R., Wolkin, A., Angrist, B., Rotrosen, J. and Paselow, E. (1988) 'Serial [18F]-N-methylspiroperidol PET studies to measure changes in antipsychotic drug D_2-receptor occupancy in schizophrenic patients', Biol. Psychiat. 23, 653-663.

Vaalburg, W., Beerling van der Molen, H.D., Reiffers, S., Rijskamp, A., Woldring M.G. and Wijnberg, H. (1976) 'Preparation of carbon-11 labeled phenylalanine and phenylglycine by a new amino acid synthesis', Int. J. Appl. Radiat. Isot. 27, 153.

Wolkin, A., Barouche, F., Wolf, A.P., Rotrosen, J., Fowler, J.S., Shiue, C.Y., Cooper, T.B. and Brodie, J.D. (1989) 'Dopamine blockade and clinical response: evidence for two biological subgroups of schizophrenia', Am. J. Psychiatry 46, 905-908.

Wong, D.F., Wagner, H.N., Larry, E.T., Dannals, R.F., Pearlson, G.D., Links, G.M., Tamminga, C.A., Bronssolle, E.P., Ravert, H.T., Wilson, A.A., Toang, J.K.T., Malot, J., Williams, J.A., O'Tuama, L.A., Snyder, S.H., Kuhar, M.J. and Gjedde, A. (1986) 'Positron emission tomography reveals elevated D_2-dopamine receptors in drug naive schizophrenics', Science 234, 1558-1563.

MEASUREMENT OF DOPAMINE RECEPTOR OCCUPANCY: CLINICAL ISSUES

A-L. NORDSTRÖM

ABSTRACT. Using PET and D2-dopamine receptor ligands several research groups have examined central D2-dopamine receptor occupancy in schizophrenic patients during neuroleptic drug treatment. High D2-receptor occupancies have been found in the striatum which give support to the theory that the antipsychotic effect of neuroleptic drugs is related to blockade of central dopamine receptors. Studies that have been reported so far regarding the relation between drug effects and D2-receptor occupancy are reviewed. In conclusion, methods are now available to determine central dopamine receptor occupancy in relation to pharmacological effects. Such relationships may be useful for optimal clinical monitoring of neuroleptic drugs.

Introduction

It is widely accepted that the therapeutic effect of neuroleptic drugs is related to their ability to antagonize the action of dopamine by blockade of central dopamine receptors. This hypothesis has been supported by the demonstration of a linear correlation between drug affinity for central D2-dopamine receptors in animals and antipsychotic potency in patients (Carlsson *et al.*, 1963; van Rossum *et al.*,1966; Creese *et al.*, 1976; Seeman *et al* .,1976; Peroutka *et al.*,1980). Previously it has only been possible to examine this hypothesis in animal models. The development of positron emission tomography (PET) has now made it feasible to study drug interaction with receptors in the living human brain (Wagner *et al* .,1983;Sedvall *et al* 1986).

Using PET and [76Br]bromospiperone, the PET-group in Orsay examined two schizophrenic patients who had recieved 10 mg haloperidol 2 hours before the PET-examination (Mazière *et al* .,1985). The striatum to cerebellar ratio was significant decreased compared to the mean ratio in controls. Using PET and [76Br]bromospiperone, Cambon *et al* 1987 examined 6 patients treated with a wide dose range of neuroleptic drugs. Measured receptor occupancy showed a clear-cut dose-dependent saturation curve with increasing daily oral dose of neuroleptics. In 8 patients PET experiments were repeated after drug withdrawal. Normal or supranormal receptor availability occured in a matter of days.

J. C. Baron et al. (eds.), Brain Dopaminergic Systems: Imaging with Positron Tomography, 191–198.

The study by Cambon *et al* 1987 was expanded by Baron *et al* 1989 who examined 11 patients during oral neuroleptic treatment, 16 patients after withdrawal of neuroleptic drug treatment and 6 patients during treatment with depot neuroleptics. The D2-dopamine receptor occupancy was highly significantly correlated in a sigmoid-like fashion to the logarithm of the chlorpromazine-equivalent dose of oral neuroleptics. Following withdrawal, normal receptor availability occured within 5-15 days. During treatment with depot neuroleptics D2-receptor occupancy was stable over the whole 4 week drug administration interval.

Martinot *et al* 1990 using PET and [76Br]bromolisuride, examined 15 schizophrenic patients and 14 controls. The patients were given different doses of neuroleptics depending on type of schizophrenic disorder. Patients with mainly negative symtoms recieved low doses of neuroleptics. Despite a weak central D2-dopamine receptor blockade, a significant decrease in negative symtoms was obeserved. Patients with both positive and negative symtoms received "usual doses" of neuroleptics which resulted in a higher D2-receptor occupancy. D2-dopamine receptor occupancy during neuroleptic drug treatment did not significantly differ between responders and nonresponders.

The PET-group at Brookhaven research laboratories performed serial [18F]N-methylspiroperidol PET studies to measure changes in antipsychotic drug D2-receptor occupancy in schizophrenic patients and observed a decrease in the uptake of [18F]-NMS by striatal tissue in medicated schizophrenic subjects (Smith *et al* .,1988). They concluded that this decrease reflects the degree of D2-dopamine receptor occupancy by the therapeutically administered antipsychotic drug.

Wolkin *et al* 1989 used PET to estimate striatal uptake of [18F]N-methylspiroperidol in 10 schizophrenic patients before and after medication with haloperidol. BPRS scores were obtained before and during treatment. 5 patients were non-responders i.e they had a less than 20% decrease in total BPRS score during treatment. Receptor availability was estimated by the "ratio index". Posttreatment ratio index values as well as percent blockade were virtually identical for responders and nonresponders.

At the Karolinska Hospital we have now for several years used PET for examination of central dopamine receptor occupancy during neuroleptic drug treatment (Farde *et al.*,1986a; 1986b, 1987, 1988a,1989). Using the selective ligands [^{11}C]SCH23390 and [^{11}C]raclopride we have determined both D1- and D2-dopamine receptor occupancy in schizophrenic patients treated with clinical doses of classical and atypical neuroleptics. The following represents a summary of the method and results from PET-experiments obtained so far.

Methods

The study was approved by the Ethics and Radiation Safety Committiees of the Karolinska Hospital. The subjects were examined at the Departments of Psychiatry and Neuroradiology at the Karolinska Hospital.

PATIENTS

The patients satified the DSMIII criteria for schizophrenia. Clinically they were responders to neuroleptic drug treatment. They had no concurrent physical illness or medication that could interfer with studies of dopamine receptors. Patients with drug- or alcohol abuse were not included. The patients participated in the study after giving their informed consent.

DESIGN

Schizophrenic patients were examined with PET and [^{11}C]raclopride or [^{11}C]SCH23390 to determine D1- and D2-dopamine receptor occupancy during treatment with conventional doses of neuroleptic drugs. At time of the PET-experiment , neuroleptic drug treatment had reached steady state conditions. The PET-experiments were performed in the afternoon, between the morning and the evening dose. Patients who were treated with depot neuroleptics were examined at the end of an interval.

RADIOCHEMISTRY AND PET-CAMERA SYSTEM

[^{11}C] raclopride and [^{11}C] SCH23390 were prepared by methylation of the corresponding desmethyl precursor analogue using [^{11}C]methyiodide (Farde *et al* .,1988b). In each experiment 100 MBq of either radioligand was injected intravenously. The specific activity varied between 110 and 1200 Ci/mmol at time of injection. The four ring PET-camera system, Scanditronix PC 384-7B, was used to follow radioactivity in seven sections of the brain. The in plane resolution of the reconstructed images is 7.6 mm full-width at half maximum (FWHM) (Litton *et al* .,1984).

EXPERIMENTAL PROCEDURE

For each patient a plaster helmet was made. The helmet was used with a head fixation system both during CT and PET (Bergström *et al.*,1981). To optimize and standardize the positioning of the putamen, Monroe's foramen was identified by CT. A level 3 mm above Monroe's foramen was chosen as the midpoint of section 4 in the following series of CT and PET scans. The head fixation system made transfer of the positioning from CT to PET feasable (Bohm *et al* .,1986).

[^{11}C]raclopride or [^{11}C]SCH23390 was injected intravenously as a bolus during 2 seconds. The cannula was then immediately flushed with 10 ml saline. In each study radioactivity was measured by PET for 45 to 51 minutes in 11-12 sequential scans (Farde *et al.*,1985).

CALCULATION OF DOPAMINE RECEPTOR OCCUPANCY

Images were constructed for each sequential scan. Regions of interest were drawn for the putamen, a region known to have a high density of dopamine receptors and the cerebellum, in which the density of dopamine receptors is negligable. To obtain uptake curves, regional radioactivity was calculated for each sequential scan, corrected for [^{11}C]decay and plotted versus time. The theory for the calculation of central D2-dopamine receptor occupancy in vivo has been presented in detail previously (Farde *et al.*,1988b). The radioactivity in the cerebellum was used as an estimate of $C_f(t)$, the free radioligand concentration in brain. Radioactivity representing specific [^{11}C]raclopride or [^{11}C]SCH23390 binding to D2-dopamine receptors in the putamen, $C_b(t)$, was defined as

$$C_b(t)=C_{put}(t)-C_f(t)$$

where $C_{put}(t)$ is the total regional radioactivity in the putamen.

The curves for $C_b(t)$ and $C_f(t)$ were then integrated from 15 to 27 minutes ([^{11}C]SCH23390) or 21 to 33 minutes ([^{11}C] raclopride) after radioligand injection and a ratio R was obtained according to the equation;

$$R = \int C_b(t)dt \,/ \int C_f(t)dt$$

R was calculated for each PET experiment at time of equilibrium. D2-dopamine receptor occupancy during neuroleptic drug treatment was defined as the per cent reduction of the ratio R in relation to the expected value in the neuroleptic-free state. The expected value for D2-dopamine receptor binding was obtained from experiments in 20 healthy subjects (mean 3.01; SD=0.45) (Farde *et al.*,1990). This value is similar to the value of 3.04 obtained in 18 drug-naive schizophrenic patients. The expected value B/F for D1-dopamine receptor binding was based on experiments in seven healthy subjects (mean 1.96; SD 0.18).

Results

The dopamine receptor occupancies obtained from the different PET-experiments are listed in table 1. Treatment with conventional doses of ten chemically distinct classical neuroleptics resulted in a 70-89% occupancy of D2-dopamine receptors in the putamen. This finding represents strong support for the hypothesis that the mechanism of action of classical antipsychotic drugs is related to a substantial degree of D2-dopamine receptor occupancy.

In three patients treated with conventional doses of the atypical neuroleptic clozapine, the D2-dopamine receptor occupancy was 38-63%, the lowest values so far obtained. Clozapine seems to be different from classical neuroleptics also regarding D1-dopamine receptor binding. In the patients treated with clozapine the D1-dopamine receptor occupancy was high (42%) as compared to patients treated with classical neuroleptics (0-40%).

In some patients treated with classical neuroleptics, akathisia or parkinsonism was recorded in connection with the PET experiment. These patients with extrapyramidal side effects (EPS) tended to have higher D2-dopamine receptor occupancy as compared to patients with no EPS.

Table 1: D2-DOPAMINE RECEPTOR OCCUPANCY IN PATIENTS TREATED WITH ANTIPSYCHOTIC DRUGS

CLASSICAL NEUROLEPTICS

Drug	**Dose**	**D2-occupancy**	**D1-occupancy**	
Chlorpromazine		100x2	78	
Flupentixol	3x2	70	40	
Flupentixol	5x2	70		
Flupentixol dec	40/weekly	81	36	eps
Haloperidol	4x2	82		
Haloperidol	6x2	84		eps
Haloperidol	3x2	89		eps
Haloperidol dec	50/3 week	85		eps
Haloperidol	3x2	84		eps
Haloperidol	2x2	75		eps
Haloperidol	2x2	84		eps
Melperone	100x3	70		
Melperone	100+150	71		
Pimozide	4x2	79		eps
Perphenazine	4x2	76	0	
Perphenazine	30x2	84		eps
Sulpiride	400x2	78	-7	
Thioridazine	150x2	74		
Thioridazine	100x2	81	29	
Trifluoperazine	5x2	75		
Zuclopent. dec	200/2week	81	11	

ATYPICAL NEUROLEPTICS

Clozapine	300x2	63		
Clozapine	150x2	40	42	
Clozapine	250x2	38	42	

eps= extrapyramidal side effects

Discussion

Results from the present study are in concordance with our previously reported data and with the studies reviewed in the introduction (*Farde et al.*,1986,1988,Mazière *et al.*,1985;Cambon *et al.*,1987;Smith *et al.*,1988;Baron *et al.*,1989,Wolkin *et al.*,1989 ;Martinot *et al* 1989). The findings give support to the hypothesis that the antipsychotic effect of neuroleptic drugs is related to a blockade of central dopamine receptors. However, also patients not responding to antipsychotic drug treatment have a high D2-dopamine receptor occupancy (Wolkin *et al* .,1989; Martinot *et al* .,1989). Wolkin *et al* discussed wether this finding could reflect an intrinsic difference in the pathophysiology of schizophrenic symptoms. Martinot *et al* found that D2-dopamine receptor occupancy did not differ significantly between responders and non-responders. They concluded that the central D2-dopamine receptor blockade is a necessary, but insufficient condition to account for the antipsychotic effect of neuroleptics.

After initiating neuroleptic treatment in acutely psychotic patients there is a clinically observed delay before antipsychotic effect occurs. By performing repeated PETexperiments after giving single doses of haloperidol to healthy volunteers, we found that a high dopamine receptor blockade is established already 3 hours after drug administration (Nordström *et al*, submitted). These data support that the antipsychotic effect is mediated by time demanding mechanisms following dopamine receptor blockade.

An important observation in present study is that patients with EPS tend to have a high central D2-dopamine receptor occupancy. The atypical neurolepic clozapine is associated with a low frequency of extrapyramidal effects. An explanation may be that treatment with clozapine does not induce the high D2-dopamine receptor occupancy found in patients with EPS during treatment with classical neuroleptics.

The accuracy of the described method to estimate dopamine receptor occupancy during neuroleptic drug treatment needs to be further explored. Preliminary data from a test-retest study of the putamen/cerebellar ratio shows that the concordance is acceptably high between two similar experiments performed in the same healthy volunteer (Nordström *et al*, submitted).

Different experimental approaches have been used to search for putative anatomical regions where dopamine receptor blockade mediate antipsychotic effect. The limited resolution of the present PET-camera systems implies that all PET-centers so far have been restricted to examine caudate nucleus and putamen, two large nuclei with a high density of dopamine receptors. With the coming generation of high resolution PET-camera systems it may be possible in the future to study also extrastriatal limbic regions.

To summarize, methods are now available to determine central dopamine receptor occupancy during treatment with psychoactive drugs and to relate receptor blockade to pharmacological effects. Such relationships may be useful for optimal clinical monitoring of neuroleptic drugs.

References

Baron JC, Martinot JL, Cambon H.(1989) Striatal dopamine receptor occupancy during and following withdrawal from neuroleptic treatment: correlative evalution by positron emission tomography and plasma prolactine levels. Psychopharmacology 99:463-472.

Bergström M, Boethius J, Eriksson L, et al (1981) Head fixation device for reproducible positron alignment in transmission CT and positron emission tomography. J Comput Assist Tomogr 8:74-87

Bohm C, Greitz T, Blomquist G, et al: (1986)Applications of a computerized adjustable brain atlas in positron emission tomography. Acta Radiol Suppl 369:449-452

Cambon H, Baron JC, Boulenger JP, Loc'h C, Zarifian E, Mazière B (1987) In Vivo Assay for Neuroleptic Receptor Binding in the Striatum Positron Tomography in Humans. British Journal of Psychiatry 151:824-830.

Carlsson A, Lindqvist M (1963) Effect of chlorpromazine or haloperidol on formation of 3-methoxythyramine and normetanephrine on mouse brain. Acta Pharmacol Toxicol 20:140-144.

Creese I, Burt DR, Snyder SH (1976) Dopamine receptor binding predicts clinical and pharmacological potencies of antischizophrenic drugs. Science 192:481-483.

Farde L, Wiesel F-A, Ehrin E, Hall H and Sedvall G.(1985a) Quantitative PET-scan determination of dopamine-D2 receptor binding in schizophrenic patients treated with distinct classes of antipsychotic drugs. Shagass C.et al.(eds): Biological Psychiatry on Developments of Psychiatry. 7:363-365. Elsvier Science Publ. Co., New York. 1986

Farde L, Ehrin E, Eriksson L, et al (1985b)Substituted benzamides as ligands for visualization of dopamine receptor binding in the human brain by positron emission tomography. Proc Natl Natl Acad Sci USA 82:3863-3867

Farde L, Hall H, Ehrin, Sedvall G.(1986) Quantitative analysis of dopamine-D2 receptor binding in the living human brain by positron emission tomography. Science 231:258-261.

Farde L, Halldin C, Stone-Elander S, Sedvall G.(1987) PET analysis of human dopamine receptor subtypes using ^{11}C-SCH 23390 and ^{11}C-raclopride. Psychopharmacology 92:278-284

Farde L, Wiesel F-A, Halldin C, Sedvall G. (1988a) Central D2-dopamine receptor occupancy in schizophrenic patients treated with antipsychotic drugs. Arch Gen Psychiatry 45:71-76

Farde L, Pauli S, Hall H, et al.(1988b) Stereoselective binding of 11C-Raclopride - a search for extrastriatal central D2-dopamine receptors by PET. Psychopharmacology 94:471-478

Farde, L., Wiesel, F-A. Nordström, A-L., Sedvall, G.(1989) D1- and D2-dopamine receptor occupancy during treatment with conventional and atypical neuroleptics. Psychopharmacology Suppl 99:S28-S31

Farde, L., Wiesel, F-A., Halldin, C., Stone-Elander, S., Nordström, A-L., Hall H., Sedvall, G.(1990) D2-Dopamine receptor characteristics in drug naive schizophrenic subjects. Arch Gen Psychiatry 47:213-219.

Litton J, Bergström L, Eriksson L, et al.(1984) Performance study of the PC-384 positron camera system for emission tomography of the brain. J Comput Assist Tomogr 8:74-87

Martinot JL, Paillère-Martinot ML, Loc'h C.(1990) Central D2 receptor blockade and antipsychotic effects of neuroleptics. Preliminary study with positron emission tomography. Psychiatr & Psychobiol 5:231-240

Mazière B, Loc'h C, Baron J-C, Sgouropoulos P (1985) In vivo quantitative imaging of dopamine receptors in human brain using positron emission tomography and 76Br-bromospiperone. Eur J Pharmacol 114:267-272.

Peroutka SJ, Snyder SH (1980). Relationship of neuroleptic drug effects at brain dopamine, serotonin, adrenergic and histamin receptors to clinical potency.Am J Psychiatry 137:1518- 1522.

van Rossum JM (1966) The significance of dopamine receptor blockade for the mechanism of action of neuroleptic drugs. Arch Int Pharmacodyn Ther 1966:160:492-494

Sedvall G, Farde L, Persson A, Wiesel FA (1986) Imaging of neurotransmitter receptors in the living human brain. Arch Gen Psychiatry 43:995-1005.

Seeman P, Lee T, Chau-Wong M, Wong K (1976) Antipsychotic drugs doses and neuroleptic/dopamine receptors. Nature 261:717-719.

Smith M, Wolf AP, Brodie JD.(1988) Serial [18F]N-Methylspiperone PET Studies to Measure Changes in Antipsychotic Drug D-2 Receptor Occupancy in Schizophrenic patients. Biol Psychiatry 23:653-663

Wagner HN, Burns HD, Dannals RF, Wong DF, Långström B, Duelfer T, Frost JJ, Raert HT, Links JM, Rosenblom SB, Lukas SE, Kramer AV, Kuhar MJ (1983):Imaging dopamine receptors in the human brain by positron tomography. Science 221:1264-1266.

Wolkin A., Barouche F., Wolf A et al. (1989) Dopamine Blcokade and Clinical Response: Evidence for Two Biological Subgroups of Schizophrenia. Am J Psychiatry 146:905-908

Developments in Nuclear Medicine

1. P.H. Cox (ed.): *Cholescintigraphy*. 1981 ISBN 90-247-2524-0
2. P.H. Cox (ed.): *Progress in Radiopharmacology*. Selected Topics. Proceedings of the 3rd European Symposium (Noordwijkerhout, The Netherlands, April 1982). 1982 ISBN 90-247-2768-5
3. M.H. Jonckheer and F. Deconinck (eds.): *X-Ray Fluorescent Scanning of the Thyroid*. 1983 ISBN 0-89838-561-X
4. K. Kristensen and E. Nørbygaard (eds.): *Safety and Efficacy of Radiopharmaceuticals*. 1984 ISBN 0-89838-609-8
5. A. Bossuyt and F. Deconinck: *Amplitude/Phase Patterns in Dynamic Scintigraphic Imaging*. With a Foreword by A. Bertrand Brill. 1984 ISBN 0-89838-641-1
6. M.R. Hardeman and Y. Najean (eds.): *Blood Cells in Nuclear Medicine, Part I*. Cell Kinetics and Bio-distribution. 1984 ISBN 0-89838-653-5
7. G.F. Fueger (ed.): *Blood Cells in Nuclear Medicine, Part II*. Migratory Blood Cells. 1984 ISBN 0-89838-654-3
8. H.J. Biersack and P.H. Cox (eds.): *Radioisotope Studies in Cardiology*. 1985 ISBN 0-89838-733-7
9. P.H. Cox, G. Limouris and M.G. Woldring (eds.): *Progress in Radiopharmacology 1985*. 1985 ISBN 0-89838-745-0
10. P.H. Cox, S.J. Mather, C.B. Sampson and C.R. Lazarus (eds.): *Progress in Radiopharmacy*. 1986 ISBN 0-89838-823-6
11. H. Deckart and P.H. Cox (eds.): *Principles of Radiopharmacology*. 1987 ISBN 0-89838-774-4
12. W.-D. Heiss, G. Pawlik, K. Herholz and K. Wienhard (eds.): *Clinical Efficacy of Positron Emission Tomography*. 1987 ISBN 0-89838-898-8
13. G.B. Gerber, H. Métivier and H. Smith (eds.): *Age-related Factors in Radionuclide Metabolism and Dosimetry*. 1987 ISBN 0-89838-953-4
14. K. Kristensen and E. Nørbygaard (eds.): *Safety and Efficacy of Radiopharmaceuticals 1987*. 1987 ISBN 0-89838-986-0
15. C. Beckers, A. Goffinet and A. Bol (eds.): *Positron Emission Tomography in Clinical Research and Clinical Diagnosis*. Tracer Modelling and Radioreceptors. 1989 ISBN 0-7923-0254-0
16. M. De Schrijver: *Scintigraphy of Inflammation with Nanometer-sized Colloidal Tracers*. 1989 ISBN 0-7923-0272-9
17. Ch. Kessler, M.R. Hardeman, H. Henningsen and J.-N. Petrovici (eds.): *Clinical Application of Radiolabelled Platelets*. 1990 ISBN 0-7923-0729-1
18. H.J. Biersack and P.H. Cox (eds.): *Nuclear Medicine in Gastroenterology*. 1991 ISBN 0-7923-1074-8
19. R.P. Baum, P.H. Cox, G. Hör and G.L. Buraggi (eds.): *Clinical Use of Antibodies*. Tumours, infection, infarction, rejection and in the diagnosis of AIDS. 1991 ISBN 0-7923-1424-7

Developments in Nuclear Medicine

20. J.C. Baron, D. Comar, L. Farde, J.L. Martinot and B. Mazoyer (eds.): *Brain Dopaminergic Systems: Imaging with Positron Tomography.* 1991
ISBN 0-7923-1476-X

21. M.K. Dewanjee: *Radioiodination.* Theory, Practice, and Biomedical Application. 1991
ISBN 0-7923-1491-3

Kluwer Academic Publishers - Dordrecht / Boston / London